I Love This Diet!

Practically Painless Weight Management

by

Arleen J. Watkins, D. Ed.

The cardiologist's diet: If it tastes good, spit it out."
— *Unknown*

I Love This Diet !

Practically Painless Weight Management

by
Arleen J. Watkins, D. Ed.

Cover Design and Illustrations by
Arleen J. Watkins

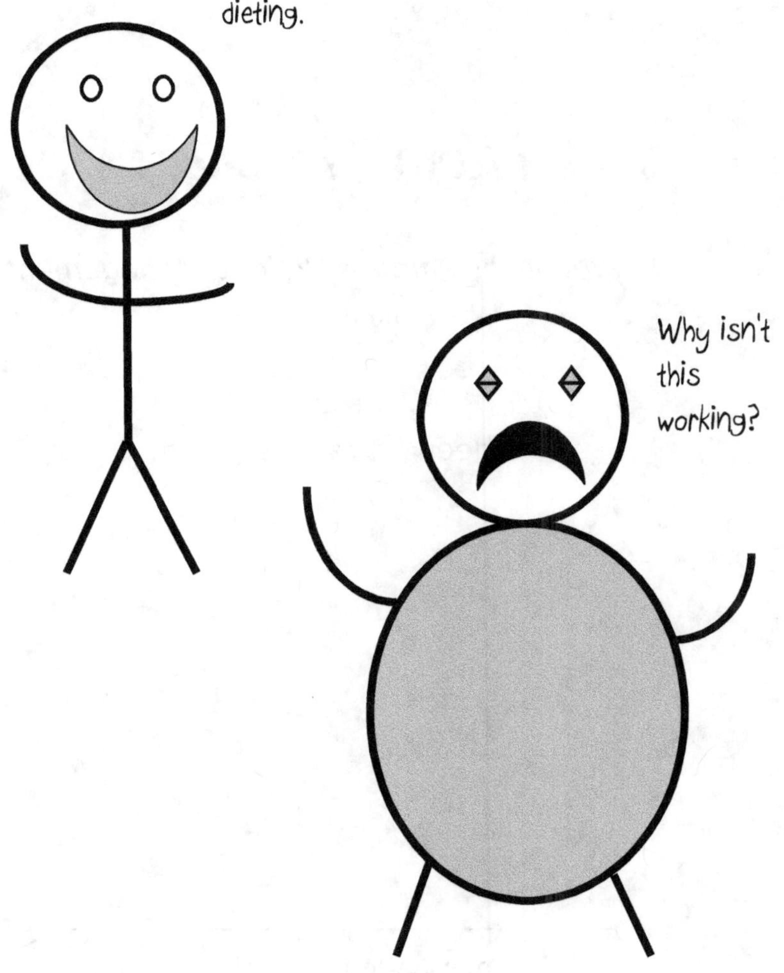

This is what I want to look like the day after dieting.
Why isn't this working?

Table of Contents

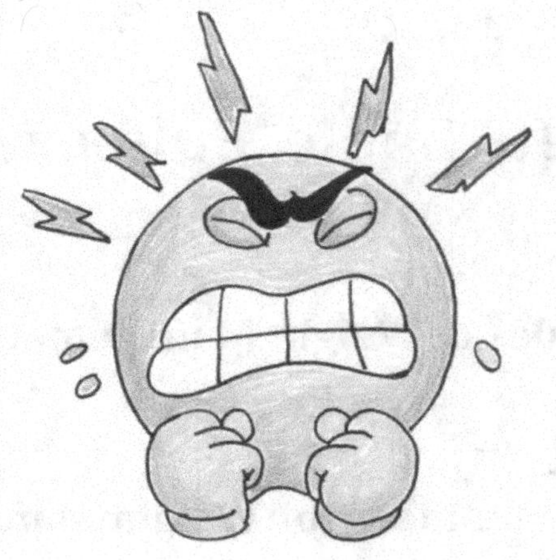

HUNDREDS OF YEARS OF
MEDICAL RESEARCH AND ALL
YOU CAN TELL ME TO DO IS

EAT LESS??

KEEP IT SIMPLE, PUL-EEZE

People ask "*Why are you writing another "diet" book?*
I say "*It's not a diet book. It's a weight management book.*"
Blank stare.
So I explain:

Diet programs are not especially effective in helping most readers *keep* weight off. The diets are low enough in calories to promote weight loss but are too stringent or complex or fussy to stick with. Diet books, even best sellers, have not completely nor satisfactorily addressed the hopeful weight-loser's need to learn to control their weight. There are still over 80% of American women who dislike their bodies and two thirds of them are unhappy with their weight. These people will most likely start their road to weight loss with a trip to the bookstore rather than to a doctor.

However, there among the promising titles they are not likely to find any diet book that will ultimately incite them to make the *lifestyle changes* necessary for permanent weight loss.

Why should this be? The bare-bones bottom-line truth of the matter is that we – all of us, without exception – like the way we live. Although we want to be able to control our weight, we want to do it without a lot of effort and we certainly do not want to make any radical life style changes. We don't want to deal with calculations and calculators, special diets, complicated weight loss plans with foreboding charts, and demanding exercise routines. We don't want to -- nor do we have to - obtain an in-depth knowledge of nutrition and physiology with their confusing terminology.

We do not want to buy expensive exercise equipment and memberships to health clubs. We may say we will, we may even embark on the path, but in the end, most of us won't because life style change is simply too demanding, difficult and demoralizing.

So what can be done? The best and most hopeful solution would be to provide the wanna-be weight loser with simple techniques that are easy to adopt and incorporate in their everyday routines, techniques that can be used individually or together. These simple techniques should not impose a radical change in lifestyle. They should, however, promote a new way to think about food, calories, energy, and activity. In the end, they may accomplish a life style change, maybe even a *radical* life style change, but only by slipping it in unsuspectingly by the back door, so to speak.

Diet books generally muddy the water with nutrition charts, recipes, exercise routines and complicated explanations or tasks to be performed by the wanna-be weight loser. The focus in this book is for those who want to lose 10, 20, maybe 25 pounds or keep their weight from creeping ever upward without major effort and complicated calculations. *It is not generally for those who want to lose a lot of weight in a short time although these techniques would work for them also - if they have the patience.*

Rationale

Therefore this book will not be a standard diet book as much as it will be a *weight management book*. While other diet books exhort people to follow certain diet plans, this book will not promote any particular diet nor provide any special recipes to follow.

This book will not render advice about adjusting the body's chemistry through diet and nutrition. It will not exhort people to get into rigorous exercise routines, nor will it promote the use of any drugs. This book will not expect people to starve themselves or make radical changes in their life styles. It will not be an exhortation about what is in our food nor will it tell people what to eat, when, where, why and how often. It will not try to get anyone to buy their food wares.

As such, this book is also not intended for people severely overweight, people with eating disorders, compulsive eaters or people whose weight is a result of medical or psychological problems.

The first part of the book will provide a practical explanation of the relationship between foods eaten and activity and show how this knowledge can be used to provide a basis for weight control. The second part will provide the reader with many ideas for easy changes in eating habits that will promote weight control. The third part will discuss other aspects of dieting including how to confront the promises of exotic diets and how to figure out if they are reasonable or even possible.

You should read this book if you want to
- *lose at least a few pounds*
- *learn how to manage your weight better*

And.....

You should read this book if you hate to diet!

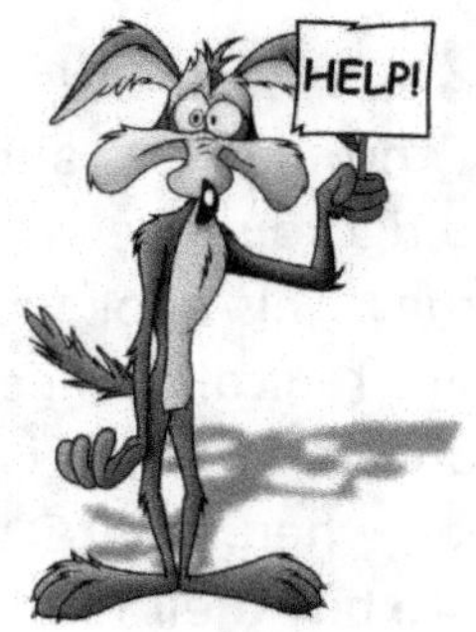

I'm still on my Yo-Yo diet.

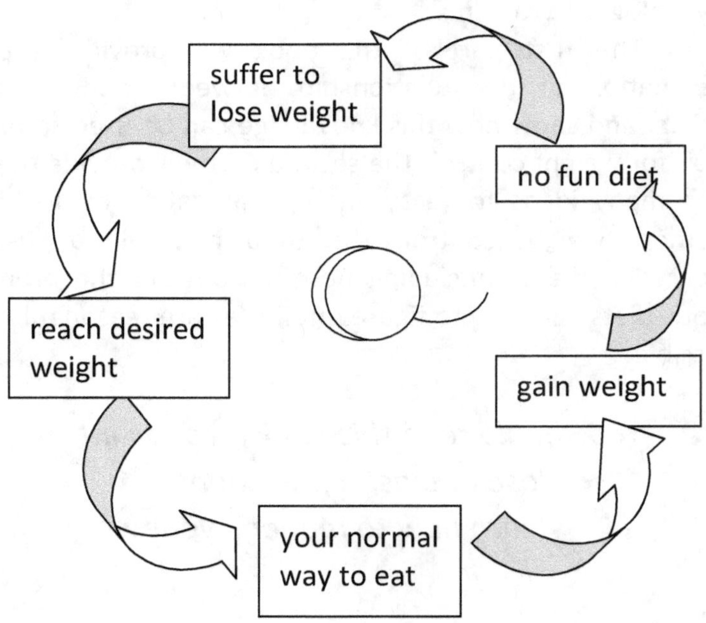

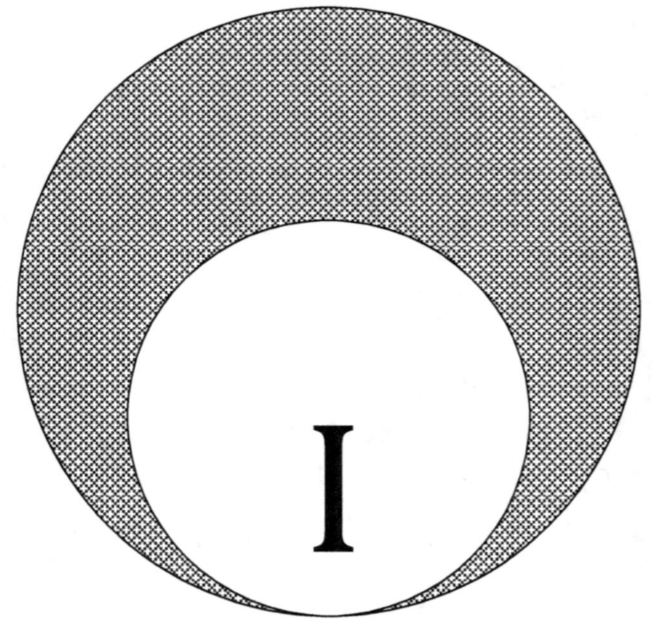

Basic Rules
for Weight Management

Do you know what I got for Christmas?
Fat. I got fat.

Thank you for calling the weight loss hotline.
If you would like to lose 1/2 pound right now,
press 1 for 18,000 times.

Chapter 1

Weight Creep

There's probably been enough written about diets, weight watching and exercise to denude every national forest 50 times over, and enough ink expended to float the Queen Mary. Everything you ever wanted to know has already been said -- and said eloquently -- and everything you didn't want to know has been said too. Despite the plethora of knowledge available in every book store and on every magazine stand, people continue to get fat. People continue to care that they get fat, try not to get fat, buy diet pills and diet plans and exercise machines and go to weight-watching classes.

On the other hand, while the public's brain is being blasted with all kinds of hi-tech information to say nothing of the guilt trips smothering their health and self-esteem, the public is being snookered into paying good hard-earned money for foods that offend the body and contribute to the problem they are trying to solve. Consequently we are, like the guy in the movie "Network", *mad as hell*.

Are you sick of being told to count calories, eat stuff you don't like, buy low fat everything and don't eat eggs or mayonnaise or peanuts or chocolate or ice cream? Are you bored with the good cholesterol-bad cholesterol debates and the saturated, unsaturated, polyunsaturated, monounsaturated, super-saturated fat issues? Are you frustrated with being told to multiply this number by that number and divide by this one to find out how many fat calories you are eating?

Do you have a hard time remembering which vitamins and trace minerals to take -- garlic, chromium picolinate, selenium, ginger, etc.-- and keeping up the newest fad on the market? Do you feel like you must carry around a nutrition book and scrutinize labels in order to know what to eat, or determine what not to eat? Do you shudder to think that if you missed the latest medical find, you might be slowly killing yourself?

Have you wondered to what extent special vitamins (organic, special combinations), special tonics, herbal extracts, beta-carotene, photochemicals, anti-oxidant-rich foods (whatever they are) -- to name but a few of the parade of items blasted at us each day – are really helpful? Have you worried about overdosing and throwing your body off balance by taking too much of some trace mineral? There are articles on both sides of the issues so how does one decide?

As for diets, have you noticed that it is not special foods or special combinations of food that make diet plans work, but that those expensive, special foods simply guarantee you will eat fewer calories per day (albeit, balanced nutritionally)? And that diets work (when people follow them) simply because they limit the number of calories a person eats?

If all these ideas have begun to confuse you rather than illuminate you, ***then you need to read this book!*** Not that all these questions and issues are going to be answered. No. Most of these issues are not even going to be addressed. Contrary to popular opinion, you don't need to know a lot of facts about nutrition or body chemistry and physiology to maintain a healthy weight. <u>What you need to know is: Why does your weight creep up every year and how can you stop it?</u>

The Marriage between Diets and Exercise

The first thing people will tell you is that you can't lose weight by just dieting, you must also exercise. That's not true although exercise is helpful and even desirable. Exercise also keeps your body toned up and fine tunes your physical system, so should not be overlooked.

Exercise can be fun, if you like to do it, but today's version – working out -- takes time and money. In the last 30 years or so, "working out" has shot up from an obscure, minor societal role confined primarily to athletes and physical fitness types, into a consuming -- and money making -- national past time.

But for some people, working out is not fun. Some people do not want to buy any stationary bikes or exercise equipment even if they are inexpensive or second-hand. Others buy them but sell them cheaply soon after purchase, hardly used. Check the flea markets, yard sales and the classified ads if you need proof.

Some people do not want to (or cannot because of lack of money or driving distance) join an athletic or health club. Work-out clothes -- fancy outfits, skin-tight stretch pants, jogging bras, special shoes, joint supports, and the like -- are expensive. Many of these items are designed for the already almost perfect body and look ridiculous on someone out of shape.

Then there are the people who just don't want to make the time to do all that exercising. They have kids and a house and a career, some friends. They don't want to feel guilty for not working out and not starving themselves with rice cakes.

Yet we all have the same basic interest: We just want to live our lives, stay healthy, and not get fat. We want to be as fit as possible without having no time for anything else -- and no money for anything else. <u>So the next thing you need to know is: How can you become or stay fit without becoming a fitness freak or going broke?</u>

New and Better Technology and Your Weight

We stop and ponder how our grand-parents and great grand-parents kept fit without our present technology and information. (For people my age, it's our parents and grand-parents!) We look at old pictures and see them relatively slim and in shape. We don't remember any talk about dieting and working out.

We reflect on the fact that in this present day we have a lot more knowledge about health, nutrition, and human physiology than they did. We realize that the people today who are living into their nineties and hundreds are not the product of our current, advanced medical knowledge in these areas. OK, in their later years these elderly people may have benefited from some of our new screening tests, medications, sanitary regulations and surgical techniques.

However, nutrition and exercise wise, they did not have our current vigilante attitude and tunnel-minded focus on health issues when they were young. Individually their knowledge about health was far narrower and inferior. They did not fuss and fret over diet and exercise, and torment themselves the way we do. They did not even have access to the health magazines, books and non-credit courses that have sprung up and entice us today from the media and market.

Today, however, health and nutrition and weight management is portrayed as complicated and difficult. We need nutritionists, weight trainers, health care experts, dieticians, resource books. We need support groups and aerobic classes and hypnotic tapes and food scales. The directives for us on how to become slender and fit barks at us from every corner of our life: TV, radio, magazines, advertisements, billboards, flyers, books, and so forth. Yet nothing works. With all our efforts, all our knowledge, all our technology, we are still overweight and struggling with the same nagging questions, the same realization that we can't fit into last year's jeans. Our children and grand children will not look at our pictures and marvel at how trim and fit we were.

Yet why should this be so? Is it because we have become more sedentary as a population, simultaneously indulging ourselves with the plethora of tastes from gourmet coffees to exotic desserts to 89 different kinds of pizza? Is it because we think we should never go hungry and so we carry food with us in cars, demand fast food restaurants on every corner & snack machines in every building, and relish "all you can eat" smorgasbords? Is it because marketers have made bigger portion sizes and added fructose to practically everything? Or have we simply bred a generation of people whose destiny it is to be fat, who inherited the genes for it, and who are physiologically doomed to carry extra weight?

The Brat Child "Drugs"

The brat child of this century is the "news" that many of us cannot control our eating habits and therefore must turn to various diet drugs to help us. We need these drugs because our weight problem is glandular, or a disease. We are *sick*! Being overweight is therefore not our fault.

As "proof" of this, we are told how simple dieting doesn't work, how people can't stay on diets, and how they gain weight back after leaving the diet. People magnify these claims when they use their own personal experiences with dieting to lend support to these "facts". Haven't they tried 15 different diet plans and failed? And haven't they starved themselves, eaten practically nothing all day or all week and never lost a gram? Don't they eat less than anyone they know?

Hence, we conclude our weight is not in our control and there is nothing we can do except resign ourselves to be overweight unless … unless … Yes, that's it! We could take some appetite or weight controlling drug. And now, because we are led to believe that we cannot control our weight ourselves, we ipso-facto become virtually drug dependent.

This leads to all sorts of other problems because no drug has no side effects eventually. There is nothing in a person's body that is not connected in some way (via nerves, blood stream, lymph system, etc.) to some other thing in the body. Therefore, a person cannot take something to regulate weight no matter where it is "focused" without having it affect something else in the body.

The inside of a body is not like the inside of a house. If you wreck a chair, the sofa still works as does the refrigerator as does the coffee pot. The only reason we can get away with treating the body so badly is because the body has an amazing determination and power to heal itself. It adjusts and isolates and seals off and discharges whatever it can. However, such marvelous activity is not without a price.

So another thing you need to know is: How can you maintain your weight without wrecking your body or becoming drug dependent.

Fundamental Questions

This book is going to address three fundamental questions:

1. How can we keep our weight from creeping up every year?

2. How can we become or stay fit without becoming fitness freaks or going broke?

3. How can we maintain our weight without wrecking our body or becoming drug dependent.

Why Should You Read This Book?

You should read this book if you want to
- lose at least a few pounds
- learn how to manage your weight better

So let's get right down to brass tacks. In the next chapter I will discuss the unalterable, formidable – but workable -- rules of the game. I will follow this with some food-activity equivalents so you can decide what you want to eat and what the consequences will be.

In Part 2 I will give you 5 "no-diet, no-exercise, no-drug" weight management tips to get you started thinking about weight management instead of dieting. Then there will be more easy tips for weight management.

In Part 3 I will discuss how to think critically about all those wonderful – but impossible – diets you read about in magazines and newspapers, and hear about on TV. I'll discuss food behaviors, illustrate concepts with analogies between the body and machines, and present a practical philosophy of weight management.

There will be a few end notes in Part 4.

Hey, my goal is to
lose 10 pounds this year.

Only 15 to go.

Chapter 2

Everything You Need To Know To Get Started!

Three Basic Rules of Weight Management

There are only three basic rules in weight management. These three rules are simple and easy to understand. However, most of us would give a barrel of dimes if we could rewrite them. You'll see why as you read on.

- **Rule 1.** If you eat more calories than you burn up, you will gain weight. If you eat less calories than you burn up, you will lose weight.

- **Rule 2.** When you eat 3500 calories more than you burn up, you will gain one pound. When you eat 3500 calories less than you burn up, you will lose one pound.

- **Rule 3.** The more you move, the more calories you burn up. Every time you move, you burn up more calories than when you are not moving

Before we go further, because these things called calories seem so darn important, let's understand and agree on what a calorie really is. We are going to need to know how to make them work for us in the context of our daily lives.

What is a calorie anyway?

A calorie is a unit of energy. The scientific definition of a **small calorie (cal)** is the approximate amount of energy needed to raise the temperature of one <u>gram</u> of water by one degree <u>Celsius</u> at a pressure of one <u>atmosphere</u>. A **large calorie (kcal)** is equal to 1000 small calories.

Foods and weight loss are actually measured in kcals, although we say calorie.

It takes 3500 (large) caloric units of heat energy to burn up 1 pound of fat. Researchers got this number by putting one pound of fat in a sealed container surrounded by water--an apparatus known as a bomb calorimeter. Then they burned the fat completely and measured the resulting rise in the water temperature.

Being Picky and Finding Excuses

Sometimes you will read in the literature things like "fat has anywhere between 8.7 and 9.5 calories per gram" like nobody really knows. The reason for this is that fat in your body may not be pure fat. The number 3500 may also be a scientifically rounded number. That means the real number is between 3451 and 3549.

The acceptable <u>rule of thumb</u> is: *fat has 9 calories per gram, and carbohydrates and proteins have 4 calories per gram.*

Little differences should not matter to you because *you are going to be managing your weight.* This means you are going to be eating a little differently every day and do things a little differently every day. No two days are ever going to be the same.

As for *burning off* calories, every person has a basic metabolic rate (BMR). Your BMR number represents the amount of energy you as an individual burn off in a state of rest per unit of time. (More about BMR later.) You do not know your precise BMR either (which can change.) One would go crazy trying to use precise numbers for both what you eat and how much you expend (that is, burn off.)

Some people in the literature mock the simple rule of "eat 3500 more calories than you need and you will gain one pound". One author proved this by pointing out that if you ate 55 calories less everyday you would have lost 141 pounds over the last 25 years. Well, if you were a 300 pound person, you'd now weigh 159 pounds. Maybe that would be a good weight for you. If you were a 150 pound person, I guess that means you would weigh 9 pounds. Ha ha, stupid us.

In real life, people do not behave that way. One day, they eat 55 calories more than they work off (caloric debt), and another day 55 less (caloric savings), or 100 more and then 75 less and maybe by the end of the month they went into caloric debt 16 times but expended more 14 times. Maybe they went into caloric debt 25 times but just a little bit, and the other 6 times they expended a lot.

It's a pretty good bet too that people are smart enough to know when to stop a deficit pattern and go into maintenance mode where the difference between energy taken in and expended every week or every month is basically zero.

You cannot let yourself get tied up in a myriad of issues and lose your focus. If you find yourself doing that, ask yourself if you really want to lose weight or are just looking for an excuse for why you won't.

In the meantime, we are going to use the scientific definition of calorie, and our rule of thumb.

The Relationship Between Activity and Diet

The relationship between activity and diet can be simply illustrated. Here are some examples:

1. If you eat the exact same thing on Monday as you do on Tuesday, but on Tuesday you lay on the couch half the day and watch TV, then you burned up more calories on Monday because you moved more.

2. If you do exactly the same activities and eat the same things on Monday and Tuesday, but on Tuesday you eat an <u>extra</u> piece of cherry pie (or potato chip or glass of wine), you will have taken in more calories on Tuesday than on Monday.

3. When you eat enough <u>extra</u> pieces of cherry pie or potato chips or wine or anything else (even celery) to equal 3500 calories over what you burn off, -- whether over the course of one day, one week, one month or one year -- you will be one pound heavier. **Period.**

I emphasize again: <u>To gain weight we must take in more calories than we expend.</u> That is, we either eat too much for what we do, or we don't do enough for what we eat. It follows that if we don't want to gain weight, we should a) eat less or b) move more or 3) tada! do both! But this you know. This is not earth-shaking news. It is perhaps sad news, but it is not new news.

What Makes Dieting So Difficult?

* Dieting is difficult when we try to severely limit our intake of food each day or we eat things we really don't like -- potatoes without butter, chicken salad sandwiches without mayonnaise (yuk), raw onion sandwiches. We are always yearning after foods we can't have, secretly waiting for the time

we can have them again. This keeps our mind on food and makes us go around hungry and uncomfortable and makes us grumpy. Eventually we get tired of it, hate it, resent it, think losing weight isn't worth the energy. The days ahead seem endless and the hill to skinny-ville gets steeper every day. If we stumble just a little, well, that's it. We're done. Hang it up.

*   Dieting is also difficult when we try to use frequent and rigorous exercise to work weight off when we have never been very active. Our muscles get sore and hurt. The exercise becomes tiring and boring and doesn't bring fast results. Furthermore, we replace fat by muscle and that can increase our weight. Discouraging!

*   Sometimes we want to eat more so we use the activity to justify our eating more. That is, we say we've burned up some extra calories in exercising, so we can have that donut or piece of pie. The trouble is, many people have no idea how the number of calories in foods compare to the number of calories one burns off in an activity. Hence, many people sabotage their efforts at weight loss by treating themselves too generously. Since they eat more calories than they exercise off, they gain weight instead of losing it. Another bummer.

*   Weight management is difficult because it requires self-discipline. We live in a generation of instant gratification. Unfortunately, a person can't be overweight today and skinny tomorrow (just as -- fortunately -- a person can't be skinny today and overweight tomorrow!)

In the end, it is best not to make losing weight a horrendous task. Since no one became overweight overnight, no one should expect to become skinny overnight. Putting on weight was slow and easy, so taking it off should be slow and easy. If you determine to lose weight by changing the habits that lead you to gain weight, then you will be able to use these same habits and skills to maintain your weight when you arrive at your destination weight.

Take It Off, Take It Easy

Weight loss and weight management is best accomplished by making a little effort every day – similar to how they tell us to walk just a little every day. Learning to manage your weight is just like learning any new skill: the more you practice, the better you get and the easier it will be. The better you get at it, the more control you will have over your life. The more control you have over your life, the better you will feel physically and emotionally. You will like moving around more, feeling more chipper. You will even begin to like eating less and like the lighter, not-so-rich foods. When you hit this plateau, you won't be expending effort to lose weight anymore.

The idea is to make small easy changes. In this way you chisel something out of your diet without feeling chiseled yourself. It doesn't have to be that whole piece of pie that you love. Just half of it. Or you can add some new activity that you like and not feel compulsive.

This is called WEIGHT MANAGEMENT.

My diet has me avoiding all fried foods
.... which is why I'm so happy that pizza is baked

Chapter 3

Weight Management

Weight management is basically creating a balance between energy in and energy out. Weight management is being aware of how much energy you need to take in (in the form of food) for the kind of activity you normally do (energy expended) and being careful to keep them about the same.

Food and Activity Combinations

I am going to talk about managing weight at its basic lower level. I've looked into the book stores and I see you can easily find books that tell you how many calories are in a hamburger or slice of pie. You can also easily find books that tell you how many calories you will burn in a 10 minute jog or a 20 minute swim.

But, wouldn't it be nice to know how much a cookie would cost you in terms of activity? For example, how far do you have to run and how fast to burn off a McDonald's hamburger. How many miles do you have to bike to burn off a piece of cheese cake?

If you buy a bag of potato chips, you know how much money it will cost you. Now, in actuality, you just bought a bunch of calories. How much energy will it cost you to burn them off?

These things are good to know. Therefore, I am going to give you a list of food-activity combinations. When you reach for some piece of food like even one French fry, you should know the level and length of activity you will need to do to burn off those calories. Then you can decide if you want to trade the food for the activity. Because that is what weight management comes down to – a tradeoff between energy in and energy out.

Please note that I am not advocating "no exercise" although in the strict sense of the word it may seem that I am. I believe exercise, i.e., working out, has come to have a certain "yuppie" meaning. It has become something *extra* to do, something to tell people you do, and you prove it by showing off your athletic club membership or your expensive aerobic outfits or your stationary bike. Ever since the marketing world manipulated us into advertising their products by wearing their brand names on the outside of our clothes or sneaks ….er, running shoes, exercise took on a new aura and became an activity associated with the middle to upper classes.

I am suggesting that you increase your activity within the normal everyday things that you do. I am also going to suggest that whenever possible you spread your activity out over the day and not throw it at your body in heavy doses and large chunks after long spaces of inactivity. In addition I will propose ways for you to manage your weight without changing your basic lifestyle, if you don't want to.

Definitions, Classifications and Ground Rules

There are a few concepts that should be discussed because they affect the way exercise relates to weight loss. For this reason I will provide some background, definitions, classification and ground rules.

- First, everyone has a different metabolism and a different body mass. The calories expended for certain activities – especially weight-bearing activities - will necessarily vary by individuals. This is because in a weight-bearing activity (like walking or running) the body is transported during the activity. The larger the body, the more energy is needed to move it or lift it. The more energy needed, the more calories expended. In broader terms, a heavy person will expend a substantially greater number of calories while walking than a thin person will expend going on the same walk at the same rate. (Of course you can up your calorie burn a bit by wearing a backpack carrying 5 or 10 pounds of something, or carrying weights.)

• Second, everyone has a unique amount of energy needed to maintain their vital body functions. The number defined to specify the amount of energy an individual needs to simply live at the most basic state is referred to as the basic metabolic rate (BMR) or the resting metabolic rate (RMR) – basic metabolism at complete rest. This number represents the smallest amount of calories one needs for respiration, circulation and maintaining vital cellular activity. This energy is proportional to the surface area of the body. Hence, the bigger a person is, the higher the BMR. By and large, men have a higher BMR than women. Also as people get older, their BMR usually decreases. The differences by age and by sex are largely due to variation in lean body mass.

• Third, it is important to remember that, *from an energy standpoint,* a calorie is a calorie is a calorie. The food source is not an issue. Three hundred calories of pizza is no more fattening than 300 calories of celery. This is because a calorie is a *unit* of heat only, regardless of the food source. On the other hand, the energy value of any food is represented by the amount of heat needed to burn it off. The caloric value of food should not be confused with the _gross energy or amount of heat liberated by the oxidation of that food_.

What confuses people about fats is that fats have about twice the *gross energy* of carbohydrates and proteins per gram. This means that we only need about half the number of <u>grams</u> of fat as carbohydrates or protein to generate the same amount of *gross energy.*

Put more simply, as a ball park figure, we can eat twice the amount by weight of carbohydrates or protein as the weight of fats for an equivalent amount of energy. Or, another way to look at it, we can only eat half as much food if we want to get our energy through fats only. And since we like fats so much, another bummer.

• Finally, the *average* daily energy expenditure of calories for women ages 15 to 50 is 2000 to 2100 calories. The average daily expenditure of calories for men aged 15 - 50 is 2700 to 2900. (More later on this.) These numbers are affected by the individual's physical activity level. That is, the more active a person is throughout the day, the higher the average daily expenditure of calories will be.

Notice that I am not suggesting anywhere that people should not use a legitimate diet program, especially if they are trying to lose a lot of weight. When planning a major weight loss, it is important to have good nutritional guidelines and a good support group. I just want you to understand that their prescribed diets are going to regulate your caloric intake. This is because the only way you can lose weight is by caloric management, regardless of the foods you eat. You can exercise and that is good, but I don't believe anyone has ever lost much weight by exercising alone. So my suggestion is that, for major weight loss, you choose a diet plan you like and one that provides good nutrition and then commit to it. About two pounds a week maximum. Any legitimate diet plan has to work.

Calories Eaten and Calories Burned

We cannot ignore the connection between what we eat and what we have to do to work it off. Every food has a caloric aspect as well as a nutritional one. Every activity has a caloric expenditure associated with it. What we constantly need to determine is: <u>What do I have to do to burn up the calories in a certain piece of food I want to eat.</u>

For example, let's consider a chocolate chip cookie. Suppose there are about 100 calories in a small rather uninteresting dry chocolate chip cookie. From my research I found that a 130 pound female has to walk briskly (4 miles per hour on level ground) for 17.5 minutes to burn off 100 calories, or this cookie. However, if she decides instead to sit on the sofa and watch the news on TV, then it will take her about 83 minutes to burn it off. Yes, that's right! It will take one hour and 23 minutes of sitting for her to burn off that cookie.

This means you can balance your calories by eating the cookie and walking briskly for 17.5 minutes, or you can skip the cookie. Let me make a suggestion. Walk first. See if you still want the cookie after you earned it. Walking can be enjoyable, but it is a little inconvenient to have to walk 17.5 minutes for a 100 calorie cookie.

On the other hand, if you would rather have the cookie and not eat anything else for 83 minutes, think about this: How many times have you eaten just one chocolate chip cookie? Two cookies will cover almost three hours. If calories were money in the bank, and cookies were a check, would you have enough money left in the bank to get you from lunch to dinner?

This is to say nothing about the fact that today's large yummy chocolate chip cookies are worth much more than 100 calories compared to those little dry ones. Some are worth as much as 500 calories!

Manage Your Weight like you Manage Your Finances

The approach I am going to use often in this book for weight management is similar to the one you use for managing your finances. Every time you put food into your body will be likened to taking money out of the bank. By analogy we could say one calorie is one dollar. As an average woman between the ages of 15 and 50 years, you have about $2100 in the bank. Every time you eat something you have to pay for it by taking money out of the bank. If you take out more than $2100, then you either have to make a deposit (through exercise) or you go into debt. When your debt reaches $3500, your debt will be cancelled but you will be one pound heavier. That is, you will be bankrupt but you can start over. You can start over as many times as you like, but each time you start over you will be one pound heavier.

If you get tired of this, you will have to figure out ways of not using so much money out of the bank because it is hard to replace. You will have to try to find ways of making deposits that are easier to earn. You might start by going to garage sales and flea markets to find bargains. That is, you could take a more serious look at lower calorie foods. You could start being satisfied with less fancy items, dresses without so many frills, cars without extras. That is, you could stop putting all that butter and sour cream on those potatoes, and creaming those veggies. You might stop buying gadgets for the sake of gadgets. That is, you might eliminate the potato chips and candy bars. If you truly want to manage your weight, you must do whatever you have to do so that you live within your budget. Otherwise, you can increase your budget by finding another job so you can earn those items you can't give up. That is, you can add some moderate exercise to your weekly routine – swimming, walking, bowling, whatever.

Pssst. . . .If no one sees you eating it,
it doesn't contain calories.

My heart says chocolate and wine
but my jeans say,
for the love of god, eat a salad.

Chapter 4

You Need a Plan

Generally, people tend to do the same things each day or over the week. What you want is a picture of how much activity you expend doing typical things so you can see how much energy you need to maintain your weight. Then, if you want to lose weight, you could eat less (or eat differently!) or become more active or both.

Research indicates that only about 50% of adult Americans engage in physical activities requiring expending energy much above the resting level. Furthermore, most everyday tasks require only a moderate amount of energy, less than three times the energy one expends at rest. And what about you?

Construct Your Own Activity Profile

It's a good idea to know how many calories you usually burn off each day before you start a diet. You need to know your starting point and you goal so you can make a plan. There are several ways to do this.

The tiring, boring, complicated way; . . .

One thing you can do is track every activity <u>you</u> do on a typical day and the <u>minutes</u> you usually spend on them. (Remember the total minutes must add up to 1440.) Multiply the number of minutes spent in each activity by the number of calories each activity burns. (Get the caloric numbers from a book or online.) Add them up. This number represents the number of calories you need to maintain yourself each day. This is an important number because you will be using it to determine if you are taking in too many or too few calories each day to maintain yourself. This number will not be an exact, granite-caste number because your activity varies each day, and also it will depend on how true your estimates of activity represent your typical day. You can get an even more accurate number by carefully loging _all_ your activities over _several_ days, and following the same procedure. Lots of work so let's look at other methods.

The technological way. . . .

You can go to a website like AthleteinMe.com where you enter your weight and check the activity and the number of minutes you will do it and the program will calculate the numbers of calories you will burn off for you. If the website asks for your age and height too, all the better. There are applications similar to this for your smart phone also.

On the other hand you could just buy one of those Fitbit watches that record everything you do and all you have to do is just look at it to find your calories burned (providing you wear it continually). How hard is that? Scary though. You'll probably find you didn't burn off as many calories as you thought.

The easy, generalized, NAP way. . . .

Now if you don't want to do any of the above to construct your own profile (boring) or buy a Fitbit watch (expensive), you can use numbers universally accepted and published in all types of legitimate health media - books, magazines, newspapers, TV programs etc. for the average person. While there is no real average person, there is a national "average person" (**NAP**) to which real people like you and me are compared when talking about calories and weight management.

The **NAP** has an occupation somewhere between sedentary and moderately active. He/she participates in some recreational activity like golf, swimming, tennis on the weekend. The female NAP aged 15 - 50 maintains her weight, whatever it is, at the same number of pounds on about 2000 to 2100 calories per day. If she's over 50, it's about 1800. The male NAP maintains his weight, whatever it is, at the same number of pounds on about 2700 to 2900 calories per day. If he's over 50, the magic number is 2400. The numbers differ in sexes mostly because of body mass.

Shocking Results...

The first thing you are going to notice looking at your profile is that you do not have a heck of a lot of calories to have fun with. Right away a wave of guilt flew over you, right? Are you thinking about that 725 calorie 3 pancake breakfast or that 750 calorie McDonald Double Quarter Pounder with cheese you just woofed down in less than 5 minutes? Or that 460 calories Starbucks Java Chip Frappe with whipped cream, you just treated yourself with after shopping? (*From Table 1 on page 39*) Yes, you are right. This is a quarter to half your daily calorie budget. In finances, this is what is known as champagne taste and a beer pocketbook.

When you spend more money than you have, you go into debt. You borrow money against another day (pay on credit card), and you pay interest. For a lot of people this debt creeps bigger and bigger and sometimes ends in bankruptcy.

Think of weight management in the same way. You have a calorie budget. After you spend your allotted calories, you start borrowing calories against the next day. Keep doing this and sooner or later, you'll be a pound heavier, then two pounds and so on. Then one day you can't button your pants. People might not notice if you are spending beyond your financial budget until you are destitute and see you sleeping under the bridge, but everyone will notice early in the game when you are spending beyond your calorie budget.

Your *really tiny calorie budget* has to be managed very carefully. A person who wants to maintain their weight - or lose weight - must be very jealous of every calorie put into their body every day. Every calorie should be high quality and efficient. You can mess up and go overboard occasionally but not every day. Even a few *extra* potato chips at 6 to 7 calories each *every day* will not get you a slender body. In fact, if you ate 3 potato chips over your calorie budget every day for a year, you would have accumulated 21 times 365 = 7665. Horrors! That's 2.2 pounds! (For some things you need to make yourself a rule that if you can't eat just one, don't eat any.)

Perhaps the solution, you think, is to increase your calorie budget. Good idea! Become more active. Maybe take a swim. 15 minutes. That should do it. But you don't know how many calories you burned off in that swim. You guess, incorrectly, that you can eat a piece or two of pizza in exchange for the swim. So if you weigh 140 pounds, you in fact put more calories into your body (at least 300) than you expended (120). Boing! You worked out and are gaining weight anyway.

<u>The moral of this story is that you cannot exercise your way out of a bad diet</u>.

So, You Need a Plan!

Probably the easiest way to start is to not think about dieting at all. In general, diets have your head thinking all the time about things you can't eat that you want, or things that you have to eat that you don't like or want. All day long you are thinking "diet, diet, diet" or "no, no, no" or "not that", or "not now." All week you are jumping on and off the scale, and feeling guilty about every extra bite. It's miserable. It's like going into confinement. No wonder dieters are grumpy and eager to get done so they can get back to eating what they want.

Ah, that last thought, sigh. Therein is the problem. Dieters gained weight with that old diet and now they are looking forward to going back to it. It didn't work before and it is not going to work now. Something has to change, yet dieters seem to be stuck between two choices: be on that horrible diet or gain weight. It's a miserable yo-yo life.

What I am suggesting you do instead is make a change that doesn't keep kicking you in the butt. How can you eat everything you like whenever you want it and still maintain your weight. There is a solution! It's very simple. Eat less. Yes. You can eat everything you like, you just can't eat *all* of everything you like. You do not have to give up any particular thing. You just have to *give up a little* of any particular thing.

This is called WEIGHT MANAGEMENT.

If you have a lot of weight to lose and want to lose it fast, then you may want to start with one of the legitimate diet programs advertised on TV or elsewhere. They definitely work IF you follow them. Any legitimate diet will always have you eating fewer calories than you are burning off. It will also try to keep you nutritionally balanced and physically fit. (Beware of those which promise more than 2 pounds a week, 8 pounds a month. These are generally not healthy for you.)

What I fear with these diet programs is that the foods and regiment will be expensive and boring, so when you reach your goal, you will desperately want to get out on your own and you'll go back to your old diet which got you in trouble in the first place. So at this point you definitely need a plan. I can 100%

guarantee that your old way of eating without a plan will do you in just like it did the first time. **A weight management plan is what you will need.**

On the other hand, if you are not in a hurry to lose that weight, you can creep your weight down just like it crept up with less effort using weight management. You can get out of the weight -war prison and get a freeing new lifestyle.

Susy: I took 30 pounds off in 15 weeks
using the "Melt-me Quick" plan.

Harry: I took $30,000 off 15 people
using my "I'll Diet For You" plan.

Chapter 5

Finding Help to Design Your Plan

Charts and the Internet

I have looked at hundreds of charts to find one to include here for you so you could make some quick and dirty decisions about what to do with that cookie and what will happen if you eat it. Unfortunately these charts are not as informative as they should be. We know everyone metabolizes differently according to sex, height and weight if nothing else. Yet these charts rarely tell you what kind of person they are talking about. It is then hard to compare numbers across several charts. Furthermore most of them do not tell you how they got the information to put on their charts. Some reference other tables, and some do not even do that.

Some charts do complicated things. Some convert their information into MET's (Metabolic Equivalents). Then they divide activities into different MET values. How is introducing a new concept helpful? Some charts tell you how to convert an activity into a number of steps and differentiate between moderate and high intensity activities. I wasn't able to figure out how this simplifies anything.

Then some charts tell you how many minutes you need to do a certain activity to burn off 500 or some other number of calories. They may even differentiate among people of different weight. But the list of activities usually consist of many things most people never do, like boxing and rollerblading. I guess the suggestion is that you might introduce one of these activities into your exercise routine. One thing we do learn from their list of activities, however, is that it takes a lot, lot, lot of work, a super lot of energy to burn off a few calories.

Exercise charts always tell you in some crude way the number of minutes a person needs to do an activity to work off some number of calories. Remember, you will burn off some calories in that time even if you do nothing! They don't tell you how many additional calories you will burn off doing that exercise. Wouldn't you like to know that? Suppose some exercise you hate doing only burns off 60 more calories in an hour than watching a ball game on TV. Then, maybe you don't want to do that exercise.

It is not enough to know how many calories are in the food you eat. It is not enough to know how many calories an exercise will burn off. *What is missing is <u>how long</u> it will take to exercise off the number of calories* in that cookie or slice of pizza or potato chip. You are trading a part of your life to do something you don't want to do for the sake of that 15 seconds of pleasure eating those 2 or 3 potato chips. It would be good if you actually memorized a few of these things with an activity length so you are always aware of what you are doing. For example, a 120 pound person needs to swim laps for a minute to burn off one potato chip!

Even when a chart tells you how many calories are in a cookie, you do not know what kind of cookie they mean, or the size, and how much sugar and shortening went into making it. You need to have information on the particular item you are consuming - it's size and composition for example. How much sugar and shortening are in it? You will notice in some tables a chocolate chip cookie is 100 calories, in others it is 500. Which one are you eating? How do you know? Any information you can get from the packaging itself will be the most accurate (and will be a surprise).

It is not that manufacturers intend to deceive, or that they are ignorant. The whole connection among exercise, calories, and food energy is simple to understand, but because the way each person is affected by health, weight, height, metabolic rate etc, there is no one standard person like there is a 12 inch ruler by which to measure. In addition foods vary in composition - sugars, fats, carbohydrates - even among all sugar cookies let alone different types of cookies and then cakes, pies etc etc etc. Then there are the different procedures for collecting data and different "people samples" from which data is gleaned. Therefore a fixed, standard table that works for everyone *exactly* can't be created. To do so, all these nutritionists and scientists would have to get together and define things the way a calorie is defined. Then all the manufacturers and marketers would have to agree to put this information on their packages. Good luck with that thought. (And make a mistake, 1000 more lawyers needed.)

So one works with statistical averages. But this is nothing new. Very few things are known in concrete. How many miles per gallon does your car get? How many people support a certain political candidate? How far is it to Phoenix? What's the weather going to be like today? What color is your hair? What's your blood pressure? What's your risk of dying from a heart attack? Et cetera. All these things depend on procedures, times, definitions, sampling, and so forth. We are going to do the same thing - work with averages.

Look at all the charts on the internet with a cautious eye and be aware that just because it is written in a book or backed by some popular diet plan or doctor doesn't mean you can bet your life on it. However, we can draw some basic, reliable conclusions even if not accurate to an individual person. The things I put forth in this book are guidelines.

These are the rules we are going to use for weight management
<u>because</u>
<u>they are</u>
<u>correct</u>
<u>for everyone</u>
<u>all the time:</u>

1. 3500 calories not burned off equals one pound gained. Follows directly from the definition of a calorie. (A calorie is a unit of energy. 1 Cal is the amount of energy required to raise one kilogram of water by one degree Celsius. Anything that contains energy has calories. One pound of fat contains about 3500 calories.)

2. If you consistently take in more calories than you burn off, you will gain weight; if you consistently take in less calories than you burn off, you will lose weight.

3. If you want to lose weight you need to burn off more calories than you take in.

Note that I said nothing about the person's sex, weight, height, health or anything else.

However, it is important to note here that the more fat a person has to lose, the quicker weight loss will happen and the weight loss will be from fat. The closer you get to your ideal body weight, some weight loss will be from muscle, and so harder to lose. (Pamela Peeke, M.D., M.P.H.)

Some Internet Tables

One of my favorite charts on the internet shows the number of calories burned per minute by exercise and weight. It is copyrighted (2004) by Linda Stradly who evidently has a website called What's Cooking America. I tried to contact her to see how her chart was developed and if I could quote some of it. I did not get any answer so have decided to just tell you to look at it on the internet. (Search on "number of calories burned per minute by exercise and weight.")

Briefly, why I like it, it lists many exercises and then gives you the calories burned per pound per minute. It's easy to use with a simple calculator. You pick your exercise, take the number that follows and multiply that number by your weight and then by the number of minutes you are doing that exercise. So if you weigh 130 pounds and pick an activity that burns off .028 calories per pound per minute and do it 15 minutes, you multiply 130 times (0.028) times 15. The result (here 54.6) is how many calories you burned off in 15 minutes. If you weigh 140 pounds, it would be 140 x .028 x 15 = 58.8 calories.

Another table I liked was "Food and Exercise Calorie Equivalents of Popular Foods" put out by Susan Bowerman. She gives you a list of foods, the number of calories in each, and the number of minutes you need to walk to work off those calories. But the list of foods (restaurant averages) is not long, and the numbers are based on a 150 pound person, and the only activity is walking without indicating how fast.

However, that was the type of table I wanted and I realized since I hadn't seen any table closer to what I wanted, I would have to do the impossible - make my own tables.

Chapter 6

My Tables

Table 1 is going to give you the calorie counts from some popular foods you can purchase in various large restaurants. (I put this table together from other tables I found on the internet.) We are going to assume these numbers are as accurate as we need them to be. Table 1 is a deliberately scary table because many Americans like to eat these items regularly. People who do so are overweight because they have no idea how much these foods cost their calorie budget.

I constructed **Table 2** using information from various charts on the internet. Not everyone wants to simply walk for exercise so I added a few other activities that I thought might be more relevant to a wanna-be weight loser. Also not everyone weighs 150 pounds, so it was necessary to figure out mathematically what the numbers would be for people of other weights.

Table 2 is an eye opener. It shows how many calories you can burn off in a minute doing a certain activity. If you move the decimal over one place to the right, you get a quick peek into how many calories you can burn off in ten minutes. You weigh 160 pounds and decide to jog? That's real effort! In ten minutes you burned off 125 calories. Hurray! But it's not even the number of calories in a decent cookie!

Exercise machines in the gym will tell you how many calories you are working off too. Consequently these activities are not listed here.

TABLE 1

Popular Foods	Cal	Notes
30 potato chips	200	
2 sl pepperoni pizza	625	med or lg pie?
dbl cheese burger w bacon	1250	
cheeseburger w fries	690	med or lg fries?
McDonald db quarter lb w cheese	750	
Outback St. House full rack baby back ribs	1156	
1 fried chicken breast	445	
chicken burrito	1175	
croissant sandwich w ham, eggs, cheese	475	
3 lg pancakes w syrup	725	butter?
bowl of cereal	175	type, milk, size?
lg mocha coffee w whipped cream	580	standard size?
16 oz frappachino	500	
20 oz soda (750 ml)	250	
330 ml can soda	140	
2 - 12 oz bottles of beer	300	
1 cup vanilla ice cream	525	
lg chocolate chip cookie	450	how big?
1 sl chocolate layer cake w icing	550	size slice?
glazed yeast donut	240	
cheesecake	710	size slice?
milkshake	780	sm, med, lg?
lg blueberry muffin	500	
dunkin donuts coffee cake muffin	590	
dry roasted peanuts (50 g)	295	

Table 2

Calories burned off
in 1 minute

Body Weight	120	140	160	180	200	220	240
Aquaerobics	3.8	4.4	5.1	5.7	6.3	6.9	7.6
Cross country skiing	8.9	10.4	11.9	13.1	14.7	16.1	17.9
Cycling (5.5 mph)	3.6	4.2	4.7	5.3	5.8	6.4	7.0
Ice skating	6.7	7.8	8.9	10	11.1	12.2	13.1
Jogging (6.5)	9.4	11.1	12.5	14.3	15.6	17.2	19.2
Martial arts	9.4	11.1	12.8	14.3	15.6	17.2	19.2
Pilates	3.3	3.9	4.4	5.0	5.6	6.1	6.7
Racquetball	8.2	9.4	10.8	12.2	13.5	15.2	16.1
Rollerblading	6.7	7.8	8.9	10	11.1	12.2	13.1
Rowing	7.6	8.9	10.2	11.4	12.8	13.9	15.1
Running (10 mph)	15	16.7	18.5	20.2	23	25.3	27.6
Swimming laps	7.0	8.2	9.4	10.6	11.9	12.8	14.3
Walking (3.5 mph)	4.7	5.4	6.3	7.0	7.8	8.6	9.4
Yoga	2.4	2.8	3.2	3.6	4.0	4.3	4.8
Zumba	7.5	8.8	10	11.4	12.5	13.9	15.1

NOTE: Move the decimal one place to the right to find the amount of calories burned off in ten minutes. For example 3.8 to 38.

Becoming Your Own Weight Manger

It isn't the intent of this book to give you magic numbers for everything you do and eat. What I want to do is provide a way for you to use information like this to become your own weight manager. I want you to be able to look at a food item you want to eat and start thinking about how many calories are in it, and relate that to how many calories you actually need in your day to maintain yourself. I want you to be able to look at a food item and have a pretty good idea of how long it will take to work it off, and if eating it will take you over your calorie budget. I want you to see that all exercises are hard work, even though they are needed to maintain good body condition. I want you to see that exercises do not increase your calorie budget that much unless they are high intensity and you do them for a long period of time. I want you to understand that no matter where the calorie comes from or how it works in your body, 3500 of them will get you a pound. I am sorry to say but you need to do what old timers used to call "counting calories." That's the ugly truth about weight management. It boils down to counting calories.

So your first task is to look at the listed items in Table I and their calories. Compare the number of calories listed with the number you are using as your baseline profile. Let's say you are a woman who needs 2100 calories (activity profile) to maintain her body needs. You're doing errands and decide to get lunch on the road. You pull into a fast food place and decide you'd like a cheeseburger and fries (almost 700 calories), and a milkshake (about 750) (Table 1). That's 1450 calories, leaving you with 650 calories left (if you didn't eat any breakfast). Oh darn, you had black coffee and a blueberry muffin for breakfast. Yea for the black coffee (0) but the muffin was 500 calories. It's 1 PM and you have 150 calories left in your calorie bank. If you can't finish off the day with something like 6 carrot sticks and water, you'll go into calorie debt. Or you can go to the gym and do step aerobics for and hour to earn yourself 550 calories. Then you can have a 700 calorie dinner.

The tables I generated for you (Arleen's Tables) are on page 111 in the back of this book. I put them there because the numbers are different for various weights and I needed a separate table for every person in 20 pounds intervals. In these tables you can have a cookie in your hand and IF YOU KNOW THE NUMBER OF CALORIES IN IT, you can look in your table (the one that corresponds to your weight) and see how many minutes it will take you to work it off in various activities. It would be an endless task to try to present the calories in every food item, so instead I broke the calories into sets of 10 calories up to 100, then for 200, 300, and 400 calories.

You can purchase a book or look on the internet for the foods you like to eat and eat regularly and note the (approximate) number of calories in them. A good place to start is at an internet site called "My Food Buddy":
(http://www.myfoodbuddy.com/php/foodSearchDetail.php).
It lists practically everything and gives the calories and other nutritional information. You can print it out, hang it in your kitchen somewhere you can get to it easily. Highlight your favorite foods. It won't be long till you will just know the amount of calories in the foods that you eat often.

Using My Tables

Find the food (and portion) you want, note the calories and look at the table that corresponds to your weight. Let's say you weigh 145 pounds and you want a slice of sheet cake with icing. <u>My Food Buddy</u> says that's about 315 calories. Look at the table for 140 pounds (yeah, I know, we use the closest pounds) and you see that to work off 310 calories (right, another average) by walking will take 56 minutes (for 300 calories) and 2 minutes for 10 calories = 58 minutes total. Almost an hour. Maybe you still have 315 calories in your calorie bank. Great. Or how about this? How about just eat half a slice? That would be about 160 calories that you won't have to walk off. And maybe you do have 160 calories still in your calorie bank. (Try to remember also that a slice is not more than an eighth of a regular size cake. And also some cakes are much richer than a slice of plain yellow cake)

If you do nothing and lay on the couch and watch some show, you will only burn off 58 x 1.4 = 81.2 calories in 58 minutes. (Do you see where I got the number 1.4? It is in the column marked <u>cal/min</u> to the left of the activity column labeled "lying or sitting quietly".) If you want to know how long it will take you to burn off that 315 calorie cake doing nothing, look under that activity and add 214 minutes for 300 calories and 7 minutes for 10 calories = 221 minutes total. At 60 minutes per hour, that's 3 hours and 41 minutes!!

Most people simply do not know the actual relationship between their activities and the number of calories in the foods they eat. I have seen women pass on eating the corn on their plate so they can have a piece of pie. I have seen people pop an extra fudge brownie in their mouth simply because it tastes good and practically swallow it whole, getting no pleasure out of those calories. One woman I knew dieted all week and then on Friday evening, spent all the calories she saved in dieting by eating a big greasy hamburger with provolone and fried onions and peppers. She wondered why she didn't lose weight. Another said she ate practically nothing and still gained weight. The "practically nothing" included a candy bar between meals.

It would really be wonderful if God had made things the other way around: A little activity burns lots of calories, and a lot of eating adds just a few calories. However, calories were hard to find back then, and it took a lot of time to spear a wild animal, so I guess that's the way it had to be.

You have all the tools you need to be successful. You have a brain and desire and information. If you want to manage your weight, this is how you have to think, especially in the beginning. Later as you get used to it, you will naturally just know how much you can eat of what type of food. Counting calories and not putting food into your mouth just because - works.

I just want to lose weight while staying in bed, watching TV and eating girl scout cookies.

Is that too much to ask?

My favorite food groups are:
Not good for you,
Bad for you,
Terrible for you,
And get your affairs in order.

A. Watkins

My doctor said
it's partly glandular
and partly 6500 calories a day.

                          I don't mean to brag, but...
        I finished my 14 day diet in 3 hours
                              and 11 minutes

It's getting really annoying how eating
makes you gain weight.

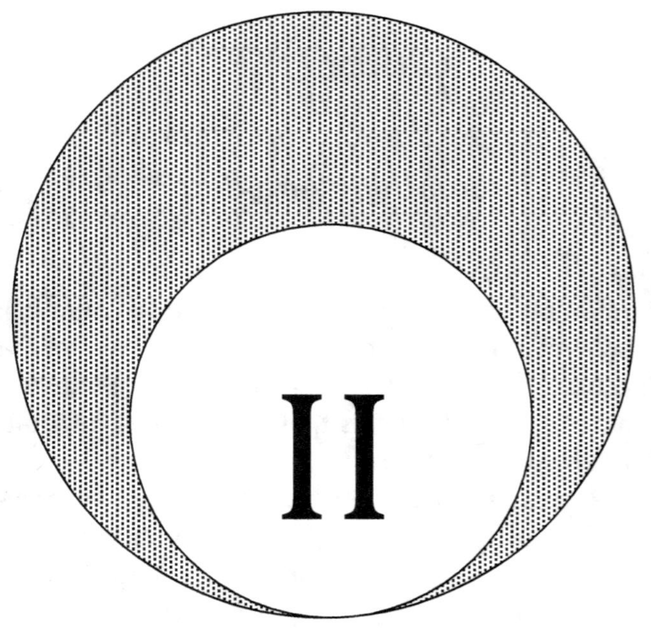

My Favorite Ideas
for Weight Management.

Chapter 7

Inching Away

Wouldn't it be nice if you did not have to count calories? And you did not have to exercise? And you did not have to change the types of foods you eat? This part of the book will give you some ideas just like this that are not very difficult to try but are very effective.

These ideas should not cause much pain or anxiety or cause attention to be drawn to you when you eat out, if you decide to use them. In fact, I recommend you just keep what you are doing to yourself to avoid getting into a position where your "friends" and relatives undermine your efforts. Sometimes airing good ideas just sets the stage for having them trampled on.

You can use as many of these ideas as you like and eschew the ones that you don't like. These ideas are especially useful for people wanting to lose just a little weight or to stop that weight gain that creeps up on us through the years. These ideas can also be useful to women facing menopause during which the body's basic metabolism rate changes.

Five Easy Ideas

Here are <u>five</u> easy things you can do to help manage your weight. With these five ideas:

- You do not have to count calories.

- You do not have to exercise.

- You do not have to take drugs.

- You do not have to change the types of foods you

  eat.

These ideas will form a basis for a philosophy of weight management. You can build them into habits that you can use for the rest of your life. If you don't read anything more than this chapter and practice it's suggestions, this book will have paid for itself in your peace of mind. Ready? Here we go!

1. Take small bites. I know. You've been told this before. You know all this information about how your mouth generates saliva and stimulates the enzymes that help in food digestion. You also know big bites swallowed whole don't digest well, and doesn't look nice either. That's all well and good. But I want to give you another reason to take small bites.

If you take a small bite, say half the size, the food on your plate will last twice as long. Now, one of the major pleasures in life is enjoying food. You can enjoy a little food as well as a lot of food. Better even. You can look at it and smell it and savor it, let it hang on the end of your fork while you talk. You don't have to be in a hurry to put it into your mouth. You are not that hungry. If you are, you should drink some water before you begin to eat. By taking small bites, you can make a little food last as long as a lot of food shoveled in. If you want to eat all the food on your plate, you will be able to eat twice as long. Besides, you can avoid being asked to take seconds because you still have food on your plate.

2. *Eat slowly.* Sure, you heard this before too. Chew every bite 50 times or something. Then it will digest better. I'm sure that's correct. I'm sure that's why you should chew food into mush before you swallow it.

But I have another reason. The reason is to keep the food in your mouth as long as possible. One of the reasons you are eating what you are eating is because it tastes soooo good. Admit it. You like it! So, let it linger in your mouth a loooong time. Really get that flavor. This is especially important when eating candy, potato chips, sweets and other high calorie snacks. You can't taste anything you swallow whole or swallow as soon as it gets into your mouth. There are no taste buds in your throat. Try it. Try keeping your food in your mouth where your taste buds are for a longer time. What do you have to lose? (Only weight!)

If you eat potato chips or tortilla chips, nibble at them. Taste the salt and the grease and the potato flavor. See how many nibbles you can savor in one chip as you watch others stuff them voraciously in their mouths. If you eat a chocolate or caramel or a small candy bar, for example, just take tiny bites and let the sweetness linger in your mouth. Suck on it and enjoy that sweet chocolaty-milky flavor. Determine to get the most flavor pleasure out of every calorie.

By eating slowly, you will find that you will not only enjoy your food much more but also there will be time for your stomach to get the information out to your brain that you are full. Right, full. Most people eat so fast, they not only don't get to taste their food, but they also get stuffed before their stomach tells them to stop putting food in their mouth. Make an apple last. Eat a muffin for breakfast? Try eating small bites over a long period of time. Do little things in between (small) bites, so that the muffin lasts an hour. Think how long you got to enjoy that muffin!

Do the same thing with everything from mashed potatoes, to broccoli, to ice cream, to steak. Everything you enjoy you can appreciate more by having a love affair with it. It's like that old saying: "Take time to smell the flowers". Well, take time to taste (and enjoy) your food.

3. *Take small portions.* Take maybe half to two thirds the amount you would normally take. Do this because then you can take another small portion if you want to. And if you don't take more food than you *want* to eat, you don't *have* to leave any food on your plate… which you might want to do if you are trying to cut down on the quantity you eat. (However, I think it is a good idea to always leave some food on your plate. It is like leaving a big tip for yourself.) Then if you also take small bites and eat slowly, you probably won't want a second helping anyway. On the other hand, if you *do* want to eat more, how wonderfully decadent to be able to take a second helping and still be within the quantity of food you would normally eat. Just remember, all the time you are eating, talk a lot and sort of play with your food as you talk. Take your time. Love it up.

4. *Drink a lot of water.* Water fills you up and doesn't give you any calories. Besides, your body needs water to flush out all the chemicals you put in it every day. Water will make your body work better. I can also tell you from experience that the more water you drink, the more water you will want to drink. Your body seems to want to hoard up the water when you don't drink enough, but when your body knows you are going to be replenishing its supply, it will use the water to flush you out and send you off to the bathroom. Never be afraid of weight gain because of water.

Now suppose you don't like water. Well, there is a way you can increase your water intake if you "don't like water" -- which some people say they don't but I think they would if they gave water a chance. One way to increase water intake is to put a splash of juice in it. Not much. This is a variation of the "lemon in the water" theme. Just a splash of any kind of juice will change the flavor and will not add many calories, but will give you a little nutrition burst. Besides, this is much cheaper than purchasing flavored water at the supermarket.

Whenever you can, replace soft drinks with water. Besides avoiding the sugar or the artificial sweeteners going into your body (and the calories), you will also avoid feeding the bacteria in your mouth that use sugar to make the acid that dissolves tooth enamel.

Whenever you feel hungry and it isn't mealtime, try just drinking water or water-aid. It will help hold you over. You'll be glad you did.

5. *Eat hard candy.* When you feel the need for a little energy, eat a piece of hard candy. There aren't many calories in a peppermint or a sour ball and this candy will be in your mouth a long time. If you feel hungry an hour before a meal, a little piece of hard candy can take the edge off your appetite and hold you over. This will be much better for you than those potato chips and cheese or a beer. Besides, too much hard candy will make the roof of your mouth sore, so you will surely quit eating candy before you have consumed too many calories this way.

Yes. I know. Many people will say that sugar is bad for you and this is bad advice. They are so sure of it that they will try to persuade you to choose artificial sweeteners over sugar. Artificial sweeteners? Are you kidding? Would you really rather harass your body with chemicals it can't use? And who knows what damage those chemicals do to your body in the long run. For all that sugar has been denigrated, a piece of hard candy is a better friend to your body than a can of diet cola.

Besides if your body is craving real sugar, it won't stop nagging you till it gets it. It knows the difference between artificial sweeteners and the real stuff. Teasing your body by feeding it artificial substances will only be frustrating, not satisfying.

Apparently you have to eat healthy more than once to get in shape.

How fair is that?

Chapter 8

More Goodies

If you just want to do things a little differently and not have to think about it, here are more habit changing suggestions. <u>Use as many or as few as you like</u>. <u>Use the ones you like the best</u>.

1. Eat more often. Like that one? Yes, but there is a condition. You must eat less each time. This shouldn't be hard because you are not going to be voraciously hungry. And if you really want to use this techniques effectively, you will eat things like fruit, soda crackers, pretzels, beef jerky, yogurt, cereal, and not things like pie, cake, chocolate candy, milk shakes.

2. Eat less. Hmmm. Not what you wanted to hear? But you see, if you want that piece of pie, then you have to eat a smaller piece. If you want a steak, ok, but eat a smaller piece. No, not a tiny scrap. Save that martyrdom for much later. Just maybe take 2/3 of what you normally would take and eat it slowly. Then really enjoy it, so you don't feel like it's a bad deal.

3. Visualize. With this technique, I try to see what the different foods are doing to my body. I imagine all the grease from those fries and that cheese getting stuck in

my veins, and all that heavy meat weighing me down. I think of all those chemicals that have to be washed back out of my body if I eat those really refined foods with all those preservatives and chemical substitutes. I try to take a look at the inside of my body and listen to how it is screaming at me not to overload it with junk. That helps me avoid things that are really bad for me.

4.   Fidget. Try pacing when you are talking on the phone, stand up instead of sitting whenever you can like when you read your mail or work on your computer, swing your arms when you take a walk, walk quickly, play with your hair, tap your fingers or feet when listening to music on the radio, do things people call fidgeting. Fidgeting can result in burning 100 to over 500 calories a day. Practically freebees!

5.   Don't eat substitute foods. OK, what this does is satisfy your craving for that genuine taste – of milk, ice cream, good chocolate, fresh butter, good soda, etc. Cakes and cookies and pies all taste better made with the real ingredients. Toast made with good bread in the morning tastes better with real butter. Salads taste better with real dressing. Pretzels – well, have you eaten one without fat? That's enough to make a person swear off pretzels forever. As for ice cream, I think most people don't know how really good ice cream is, because they are used to eating all those additives that don't even allow the ice cream to melt. There's this big blob of mush that looks like ice cream but feels and tastes like flavored Styrofoam.

When you eat those toy, fake foods, remember they are filled with calories just the same. However, they are so unpleasant, they do not satisfy you. So on one hand you put a lot of gunk in your body that the body has to work hard to use or, more likely, get rid of, and on the other hand you've used up your calorie allotment eating something that doesn't satisfy your craving and so only makes you want more of the real thing. One other thing to remember about foods made with low fat or artificial sugar: if one ingredient is decreased, the other one is probably increased. If the item is low fat, they make it taste better with more sugar, and vice versa. So, for the money (and calorie allotment), avoid as much of that as you can. In return, eat a little less of the real thing. <u>Promise yourself that if you don't like the down grade you won't eat it.</u> See if you aren't happier.

6.   You won't like this one. I suggest you cut out certain foods almost completely. Really high calorie foods like pizza, chocolate, cheese, French fries, potato chips, peanuts, ice cream and so forth *that you are not able to control the amount and the number of times you eat them,* are better not to have around. Why tempt fate? For me, I don't purchase certain items I like because one little piece is too many calories to work off. However, if I really want a candy bar, I go out and buy it. I eat what I want and throw the rest away. If I go out and there is only pizza, then I have the smallest piece and enjoy it without guilt. Generally people will not pressure you to eat more if you eat slowly and don't draw attention to yourself by saying something like "I'm on a diet." Remember whatever calories you take in, you are going to have to work off.

Eventually no-no foods will become easy to avoid, because, in combination with visualization, you will get used to not eating so much heavy grease – which is the ingredient that most people like to taste when they eat. You won't learn to not like them. It is more that you won't like the way you feel when you eat a lot of them.

7. Don't keep favorite candy around. Keep around, rather, some hard candy or some candy you can resist. Then if you really need a picker-upper in the form of candy, you can eat a little. And if it isn't a sugar picker-upper you need, you might not eat any candy at all. But if you do eat some, you will be eating it for the right reason – because your body is craving a sugar boost – and not just for the taste of it. It's always a good idea to keep candy slightly out of sight. Why keep it piled nicely on the coffee table in a pretty dish? I've gone in people's houses and taken a piece or two of some candy just because it looked nice in the dish and was available. So, dumb to tempt yourself like that in your own home.

8. Eat pretzels and crackers. When you are really hungry between meals and those hunger pangs are tugging at your tummy, eat a soda cracker or a pretzel. A few of them will fill up your tummy and eliminate those hunger pangs. You won't be able to eat a lot of calories eating them and they will even take the edge off your appetite for the next meal. In fact, before a meal, eat one or two soda crackers to cut back your hunger. This will help you if you want to cut down on the amount you eat at the meal.

9. Dilute drinks. Before you get turned off on this one, think about those fruit punch drinks you buy and that new fad "flavored water". Same old stuff with a little more water in it. Why not do it yourself and save yourself the money

at the same time? Instead of drinking a big glass of orange juice, try taking half the amount and topping it off with water. Use carbonated water if you like. You will create a fresh-tasting fruit drink with half the original calories and which will be just as good for you as if you had drunk only a half glass of orange juice. You don't have to start with half and half. You could switch to 2/3 orange juice and 1/3 water – or ¾ and ¼. This enables you to get used to a slightly different, less sweet taste, and lets your body learn to like the less sweet, less rich liquid it had been getting. In the meantime, because you are using real orange juice (or whatever is your favorite juice), you will be more satisfied and have less craving for just any old food.

10. Cut down or cut out alcohol. There is nothing good for you in alcohol. Calories without nutrients. Interferes with your sleep. Affects your family life, driving, ability to solve personal problems. If you don't want to cut out alcohol, at least cut back on one drink per social session and no drinks before you go to bed. There are about 150 calories in one bottle of 12oz beer. If you drink two bottles of beer less per week, you would cut out 300 useless calories. In 12 weeks you will have lost one pound. In one year, you will have lost 5 pounds. Just by this one act alone. (That is, if you don't eat or drink something else in its place.) Think about it. On the other hand, if it is just that bitter-beer taste you like, why not switch to non-alcoholic beer? There are only 58 calories in a can of Sharps. That's 100 calories you save every time you would reach for a beer. Of course if you drink because you want a buzz, what can I say.

11. Get a hobby and keep busy. Did you ever get really involved in something and notice how the time just passes by quickly? That is the inspiration of "time flies when you are having fun." The message here is that if you can find a hobby you like, especially one that keeps your hands and mind busy, you will find yourself having less time to nibble. When people read or watch TV, many times they have a bowl of pop corn or candy, some pop or beer, pizza, or chips and dip beside them. If this is you, this is a behavior you definitely have to work on changing because there is no way you can sit in front of a TV or with a book for an hour and work off as many calories during that hour just sitting as you are putting into your mouth. Whatever you eat is probably a major net gain of calories. This can be the hardest one for you to master, but you will have to put temptation away. It would be better for you to simply save supper until you begin to watch evening TV programs than to eat supper and nibble besides.

12. Don't eat late at night or before you go to bed. In the first place, that food is just going to lay there in your belly and affect your rest and probably contribute to fidgety dreams. However, most importantly, you are only going to burn off about 60 calories per hour while you are sleeping. If you sleep for 6 to 8 hours, that's 360 to 480 calories. That's less than one slice of decent pizza, less than a beer and 30 fries. If you are really hungry at bedtime, eat either a few soda crackers or some pretzels. That will keep your tummy from growling and provide fewer calories than you will burn while sleeping.

13. Cook as many things as you can from scratch. One reason this can work is that you can have more control over the

number of calories in a food item. You can cut back on the amount of sugar or oil called for, you can cut off fat from meats, take skin off chicken, etc. You can substitute skim or 1% or 2% milk products for whole milk and cream. You will find that you do not need to add that lump of butter to a can of soup or vegetable. If you want to spark up the flavor, you can use herbs. (Check your recipe books for ideas.) Seasoned rice vinegar perks up vegetables, and can be used for salad dressing with no calories to speak of. Tamari soy sauce is also a goody on salads.

Another reason to cook from scratch is just as important. When you cook from scratch you will not be adding all those nasty substitute ingredients, preservatives, and fake flavors. This means your will be putting more wholesome things into your body and your body won't have to work so hard to figure out what to do with that artificial junk. Maybe you body will just flush it out, but then maybe it will store it in some cells somewhere ready to start trouble sometime when too much has accumulated. Furthermore, your body will like the foods it is used to, and was made to operate on. These foods will satisfy the body's needs and will not set you to craving something, you don't know what. Your body will stay more chemically in balance and will foster health. If your body doesn't crave the nourishment it didn't get from that substitute substance, you will not be as easily prompted to reach for other food.

14. Eat vegetables. Well, you know that. You are supposed to eat vegetables because they have all those good things in them. That is true. But I want to encourage you to eat more vegetables for two other reasons. The <u>first</u> one is that your body really does need what is in those vegetables and so if you don't eat them, your body will keep asking for more food. Eventually it will get enough of what it wants from other foods including the junk foods you give it, but the price to pay will be in mega-calories. So not eating veggies can make you fat because other foods don't have enough of those good nutrients to satisfy you. You have to eat so many more of them and their high calories before your body is satisfied. <u>Second,</u> you can eat a lot of veggies for few calories. You can virtually fill yourself up and not eat as many calories as in a Big Mac. (Well, don't dump a pile of butter or cream on those veggies. I'm talking pure veggies here.) If you don't want to eat veggies because you don't care about nourishing your body properly, eat them because they fill you up on relatively few calories. You can look in a recipe book to see which veggies are best, but really, practically any veggie will do. Minus avocado and peanuts, good for you but contain a lot of fats.

15.   Don't talk about food. Don't talk about diets. Don't hang out with people who want to talk about food all the time. The more you think and talk about food, the more you have it on your mind. The more you have it on your mind, the more you will think about how good something tastes and how hungry you are. I find I rarely think about having a milk shake unless I am in the car on a hot day and drive past a Dairy Queen. Then I have been known to change direction to get one. But you see, this doesn't happen often, and it is an appetite introduced by my thoughts. Sometimes when I get there, I find they don't have the flavor I like (butterscotch), so then I don't get one. You see, I am not going to spend my calories eating something

I don't really want. My calories are precious and I am jealous of them. So I use them for things I really like.

16. Don't tell anyone you are on a diet. The first thing people do is try to undermine you. Somehow, people, especially chunky to overweight ones, do not want you to get skinny because then they would feel guilty. After all if you can do it, why can't they? So they want to prove to themselves that you can't do it. They will offer you something and when you say you are on a diet, they will tell you it's just a little piece, or someone's feelings will be hurt, or it's a special recipe or it's a special occasion, and so forth. You don't need to listen to all that. Best thing to do is just say you are not hungry, you just ate. (You can make that true by eating a piece of celery or apple before you go.) Say, hey, that does look good though, can I take a piece home with me for when I am hungry? If they say "you can certainly squeeze in a bite, can't you?" you can say "No, not right now. You just can't believe how full I am. I just finished off half a chocolate cake." It's a lie, but then they shouldn't be so pushy. Then when you wrap up the pie or whatever, you can save it for later or trash it on the way home, or you could offer it to your neighbor, or maybe give it to some neat guy or gal you've been wanting to meet.

If you are at a party, you should keep your plate filled with veggies (preferably no dips or just a little). If anyone sees you with an empty plate they are likely to come to your rescue with a high calorie cookie or something. If so, let them put one of those items on your plate but carry it around with you until you can dump it in the trash. As for drinks, see if they have sparkling water at a party. It's always a good idea to take something to a party anyway, so why not take some sparkling water and some wine, to make coolers, you say. Then you will be sure to have sparkling water when you want it. But if not, take a drink you don't want and hang on to it. Pretend to sip on it when people look at you, then dump it in the bathroom sink later. Refill your glass with water and put a straw and lemon in it. If you feel all of this is too stringent for you, then take that wine and drink a little but add sparkling water to top it off. You can keep doing that until you have mostly water. Make sure no one notices. The whole idea is to make people think you are doing what you always do, so they don't side track you.

17. Balance the calorie scale. Some products are the same but different. You look on the package in one brand and there are 200 calories per serving. For another brand there are 160. Which should you buy? Good idea to check the number of teaspoons per cup at the same time, if it is hot chocolate, for example. You might not like only 2 teaspoons in your cup, as in the 160 calorie variety. If not, you have to add in the extra calories from that third spoonful. Another thing to check is the number of calories in a serving and the size of the serving.

18. Walk with a clip. Don't just walk, or shuffle around. Don't drag your feet. We are talking movement here. Pick up those feet, move those arms. Walk briskly wherever you go. Even little moves burn up calories and help keep you fit. All this activity will increase the number of calories you will burn in that activity. More calories you burn, more quickly you lose weight *provided you don't increase your calorie intake.*

19. Straighten your shoulders and back. You will look and definitely feel better (after you get used to it). If you are used to slumping, standing straight will take energy and feel strange for awhile. But it is a way to use up more energy, that is, burn more calories. The better you look and the better you feel, the better you will feel about yourself. The better you feel about yourself, the tougher you will be on yourself about keeping on that maintenance routine.

20. Watch skinny people. See how they do things. Do they amble? Do they race up the stairs? Are they busy all the time? Do they move a lot? Do they pace even when on the phone? When they talk, are they animated? What food do they carry around with them? Cigarettes? Perhaps. Coffee? Probably. Doughnuts? Unlikely. Do they work quickly, talk fast, get ready to go places fast? Do they nibble while working? Do they stop at fast food places and buy chocolate bars? Do they gobble their food? Hey, study skinny people and emulate them. You can look like them if you do what they do. (Note: do not look at people who binge themselves and become bulimic. Forget anorexia types too. We are talking about healthy weights.)

21. Elevators! If you are only going up one or two flights of stairs, why not use this opportunity to burn off a few more calories? The idea is to lift the weight of your body up those steps. Of course it can get you out of breath in the beginning, but after awhile you will be too impatient to wait for a dumb elevator when you can whiz up those steps in 30 seconds. Some people I know pass up this little exercise and then go work out in a gym. Fine if you

like working in a gym and spending time and money there.

Another way to add a little exercise in your everyday routine is to park in the far end of the parking lot. That is, don't ride around a parking lot in front of a grocery store or where you work until you get a parking spot really close. Just park and walk. It isn't fun to <u>have</u> to park close in the handicap zone. Appreciate and take care of your health while you have it. (If it is raining, you could try to park closer, but then you could also race through the rain. Better!)

22. Wear comfortable clothes and shoes so you can move. I knew a person once who would never walk anywhere because her heels were so high, her feet would quickly hurt. She could only take baby steps in tight skirts. This meant she only walked between offices and from the car to her desk, things like that. She looked great because she dressed great. But this is the way weight begins to accumulate. Comfortable clothes and shoes do not have to be ugly.

23. Look in the mirror. What you see there is what you are. Look at your side view. Does your belly hang out? Suck it in! Do you see the lines in your underwear? Worse, can you see the cellulite in your legs through your pants? Maybe you could have a picture of you scanned into a computer and then have your body stretched fatter. You could see what you will look like if you continue to eat more than you burn off. You could put this picture on your refrigerator.

24. Don't dip it, fry it, cream it, butter it. That's all extra, unnecessary calories. Yes they make the food taste very good. That's because we like the taste of fat, and fat is the basic ingredients in these items. Just remember you can only eat half as much in fat as you do in carbohydrates and protein to release the same amount of energy. That is, 1 gram of fat produces 9 calories, but 1 gram of protein and carbohydrates produce 4 calories each. So pick. Eat fat but less food or don't eat fat but eat more food. You will really be surprised to see how veggies really taste too, without being disguised by all those creams and dips and butter toppings. You will develop a taste for not-so-rich foods and maybe even easily get heartburn or indigestion from eating excessively greasy items once you have changed your diet.

25. Don't hang around food. Better to keep all your food in a cabinet or in the refrigerator. Out of sight, out of mind. Better also not to buy more than you need at one time. Some people can't stand it if they think there is a candy bar in the house. They just have to eat it. Well, then, do not buy a bag of candy bars. If you are really craving a candy bar, get in the car, drive to the store, and purchase one small candy bar of the kind that will satisfy you, open it up and eat it as slowly as possible. If you can eat only half, great. Toss the other half out immediately. Go home and don't think about it. Just go back into maintenance as if nothing happened. Your new eating habits will tolerate a splurge or two here and there. It just can't be too much or too often. What we don't want is for you to go out and buy 5 candy bars and eat them all at once. That will use up every calorie you were able to save for a week or more. You will not need 5 candy bars to satisfy this sudden craving. Only eat as much as you need to get

through it. And don't leave the rest of it around to tempt you. What you are doing here is building new habits and new ways to think about food, and how to handle crisis situations.

26. Avoid festivals where there is a lot of food, or avoid the food vender area. There will be so many different types of food there for you to try and most of them will be laden with fat. If you do go, don't go hungry. Eat before you go and don't plan on eating anything there except perhaps for just one item that you choose before-hand. Perhaps it will be a glass of cider or lemonade. Perhaps a small dip of ice cream or corn on the cob. Whatever you choose, make it something you really like and try to choose an item that is not too high in fats or sugars. That way you will kill a craving but keep it in your control.

27. And really avoid smorgasbords. If you pay for the food — especially if it is a good price — you will tend to want to take advantage of what you bought. You will tell yourself it is ok to have an eating splurge because after all, you paid for it and that's what people are expected to do. Also the variety of foods will encourage you to take a little of everything and that will cause you to take much more food than you should eat. A smorgasbord is hard on everybody. Better to buy off the menu. (If you are a person who can control the amount you eat off a smorgasbord, then you will be paying too much for your food.)

28. The same goes for parties and potlucks where there is lots of food. In these places, the people always show off their best. This means they will have lots of fat in their foods or they will be very sweet or both. That's what

people like, really rich things, lots of double chocolate, creamed sauces and dips, potato chips, cheese cake, you name it. The food will be hard to resist. *So if you do go, you need to protect yourself with a plan.* First, don't go hungry. Second, go late. Third, be last in line so a lot of the really tempting things will already be gone, and there won't be much left of what you want for "seconds". Fourth, take tiny - at least small - pieces of the things you really can't resist and don't feel guilty about the calories in them. (And remember to really enjoy that food by eating it slowly and savoring it.) Fifth, stay as far away from the food table as much as you can. Sixth, drink a lot of water. Keep a glass full in your hand. This will give you something to do with your hands, and you can sip on it whenever you feel an urge. But also, water is filling. If you keep your belly filled with water, you won't have much room for other food. Seventh, get engaged in a conversation (anything but food) with some interesting person, preferably one of the opposite sex. This is a good time to talk about a movie you saw or a book you read. Eighth, if hassled, don't be afraid to lie and say you are not hungry or you don't like something, or you already had some item. *You* are the one who is going to have to burn off the calories so *you* be in charge – in whatever way you can – of not putting any more in your mouth than you want to. Ninth, mill around a lot and watch people. Keep busy. Tenth, leave early. Better not to help clean up anyway. Those licked fingers and that last scrape out of the bowl or the last lonely stuffed egg can add calories too. Oh, and take some item to the potluck you feel good about eating. That way you'll have at least one food you can enjoy your fill on.

29. Brush your teeth often. Food doesn't taste as good on a peppermint mouth. Also, a peppermint mouth tastes good in itself and will help you avoid putting something else in it, like food that you don't need.

30. Don't chew gum. I don't think there is anything worse than trying to stave off hunger by chewing gum. That activates the saliva glands and puts you into an eating motion. Your belly starts to gnaw, and then, that's it. You have to eat something. Suck on a piece of hard candy instead.

31. Break bad food habits. It's not the potato, it's the sour cream on top, and the butter, and cheese. It's not the bread, it's the butter. It's not the broccoli, it's the cheese sauce. It's not the green salad, it's the tons of rich dressing. Salads are not supposed to swim. And so forth. What you can do is eat less of the item. However, it is better to learn to put less goop on your food and eat the same amount. Also you can try other things. Use herbs for flavor. Try a potato with cottage cheese. Try seasoned vinegar on your salad. Try nothing on your vegetables and bread. If that isn't helpful, try half as much cheese, half as much butter. *But don't use fake stuff*. That will not satisfy you and you will only eat more trying to get satisfied. Always enjoy your calories.

32. Steam your vegetables, or microwave them. All the goodies stay inside. Vegetables will taste sweeter and fresher. If you want second and third helpings, have at it. You can't appreciate vegetables until you have eaten them steamed or micro-waved. You will not need to

camouflage their taste with rich sauces and creams. Juice your vegetables.

33. Get a really good blender (like a Vita-Mix) and eat your veggies raw. You can throw practically anything in there and turn it into a great smoothie. Fruits too and veggies, including the skins, separately or together. Add protein power or yogurt. Start with their recipes and then make your own. The biggest plus of juicing for weight loss is that it adds valuable, nutrients with a wealth of health benefits at a minimal calorie cost, and with no dietary fat. Fresh vegetable juice curbs cravings and is an healthy appetite suppressant. It also stabilizes blood sugar levels, boosts the immune system, and soothes the digestion.

34. Eat marshmallows. When you want something sweet, as an alternate to hard candy, try marshmallows. They are fluffy in your mouth and sweet and last awhile, but not too high in calories. (Do not make them into s'mores!)

35. Drink water before you go to bed. This will help you feel full and give some extra water for the body to use while you sleep to cleanse your body. (You know you are going to get up in the night anyway.)

36. Don't be afraid to leave food on your plate or throw away half a candy bar or half an ice cream cone. You go into an ice cream shop these days and they charge you $3.50 for a huge gob of ice cream. You don't want that much but there is only one size. You feel like you should eat it all because you paid so much for it. However, those calories are more expensive than the money. You are the one who is going to have to pay the piper. So again, once you are satisfied, toss the rest.

37. Try altering your recipes. You can bake a cake with less oil and sugar. You can make jelly with less sugar. If you don't like it runny, try adding some gelatin. I make orange marmalade with orange juice and I cut down on the sugar. Try substituting cottage cheese or yogurt for sour cream and other cheeses. Try Tamari soy sauce and seasoned rice vinegar on your vegetables and salads instead of dressings and sauces. Be creative. It's your health. It's your weight. You are in charge. You just need to learn new ways to manage foods.

38. Eat only when your true self is hungry. Nervousness is not hunger. Depression is not hunger. Sadness is not hunger. Frustration is not hunger. Fear is not hunger. Boredom is not hunger. Anxiety is not hunger. Got it? Furthermore you do not have to eat when you are driving, or watching TV, or reading a book, or working on the computer, or socializing with friends, or playing chess, talking on the phone, or doing paperwork. You are not going to starve. For the most part these are nasty habits. Eating is not just something to do, like twiddling your thumbs. Eating is not like putting your shoes on in the morning and taking them off again at night. Eating is more like getting a tattoo in the morning. If you want to take it off you have to somehow "undo" it. Eating when you are not hungry is calorie costly.

This salad tastes like... I'd rather be fat.

Chapter 9

More Ideas

1. Bake your own bread. Buy yourself a bread machine and see how easy it is to improve the quality of your meals while reducing calories. There is only 1 tablespoon of real butter in an entire one pound loaf. There are only good, nutritious ingredients. No preservatives and no substitutes. If you don't pile the butter on, it is really a nutritious way to "fill up".

2. Take supplemental vitamins, just in case, to make sure you are getting good nutrients. It's a good insurance policy and it is cheaper than paying dues to the doctor after the fact.

3. Do some fun activity at least once a week. Do something fun with the family. Maybe bowling or tennis. Perhaps it would be a regular walk. Some like to bike together or go hiking. Take water and fat free snacks. The activity will bring your family closer and give you some great easy, no pain exercise. That is, you won't be doing it for the exercise, but for fun and for family enjoyment and closeness. My kids and I used to walk to a water reserve nearby. One carried a half loaf of bread, another a jug of

not-too-sweet cool aid. Another carried a little peanut butter and jelly (and no butter) and maybe a hard-boiled egg. I carried an old sheet and we had a great picnic after our walk. We played tag and threw rocks in the water, picked flowers. Since there are so many calories in peanut butter, make sure you don't spread it with butter and you don't smear on too much. I also recommend you use the natural kind that is pure ground peanuts and maybe a little salt only. It's family, it's fun, it's not fattening.

4. Always dress in clothes that fit, so you look good. Don't let yourself look sloppy or it may transfer over to your eating habits. If you get sloppy there, pretty soon those sloppy clothes will fit you and then what? A new and bigger wardrobe? Come on!

5. Don't taste foods you prepare while you are preparing them. And definitely don't finish up the food on any body's plate. You have heard it said that it is the little foxes that spoil the grapes? Well, it is the little tastes and bites that spoil the diet. Keep your eating record clean.

6. Reduce fat intake whenever you can. This means more than just trimming fat off meats and removing the skin from chicken. It means cutting down the amounts of butter you normally use in sauces, icings, seasoning vegetables, on bread. (Actually, you can learn to like sandwiches without butter when you are also using peanut butter or mayonnaise or mustard because these items really provide quite enough flavoring.) It means using 2% milk in your coffee if you don't like it black, or learning to like it black. It means cutting down on the amount of mayonnaise you use in coleslaw, potato salad,

sandwiches. It means cutting down on the amount of cheese you use in sauces, serving fewer cheese sandwiches, macaroni and cheese type dishes, and putting less cheese on sandwiches, ordering hamburger straight, etc. It means eating fewer French fries, and pizza. It means eating less fried foods period. Anytime you elect to replace a meal with a lower fat version, you are doing your "diet" and body a favor. *Promise yourself to replace one fried-food meal a week with a poached, boiled, broiled or baked in foil one, and to put only ¾ the amount of butter or cheese in any dish calling for these ingredients.*

7.   Don't skip meals and don't eat less than 1000 calories a day. It is not smart to allow yourself to get too hungry or you might end up stuffing yourself with high calorie/low nutrition foods. When you are too hungry, you cannot sustain your energy and will power. Breaking down is discouraging and ruins many a person's good intentions.

8.   Buy quality foods and ingredients. We talked about this before in the section on food substitutes but it bears repeating. Good food that you like and is good for the body is eminently more satisfying so on both counts is more likely to decrease craving.

9.   Don't be an emotional eater. Don't let your moods -- stress, pain, boredom, anger, disappointment, anxiety and so forth – dictate your eating habits and run your life. Many parents have inadvertently set their children off on this path by comforting a child when experiencing a disappointment by treating the child to an ice cream cone or pizza. These are powerful habits to break and require

much self awareness and self determination. If you see in yourself a correlation between eating and any of these moods, determine to find some other activity to do in its place the next time that mood strikes. It may be to treat yourself to a movie or a drive in the country. I find walking and swimming a great mood leveler. Some people use reading or a lounging in a hot bath. (I would suggest shopping but you could wind up with an overdrawn account, so best not to change one bad mood distracter for an equally bad one.) The point is, you want to feed your body and not your emotions since your emotions can't eat. If your emotions need attention, then try to identify what that emotion is and do some creative thing to get you through it. You might need to see a counselor or solicit a friend to help. However, adding a "fat" body to a bad feel is a really destructive solution.

10. Change the way you eat. For example, besides the tips I already presented, you could: use teaspoons instead of tablespoons, use small plates and salad forks. These will make it look like you have more food, force you to take longer to eat, and make the food last longer. (This is not a favorite technique of mine because your head knows you are playing a game. Better to be honest with yourself and just do your usual but use smaller portions.)

You can also deliberately put your glass or cup or fork down between each bite to force yourself to lengthen your eating time. You could also keep all the food dishes on the stove staying warm so people have to get up to serve themselves. This way the food is not readily and temptingly seen. (This will also reduce the number of dishes to wash, always a good result in my book.) You can also drink a lot of water before coming to the table, and drink a lot of water between meals. But then we said that before.

11. Learn a new routine. If you have a coffee beak at 10 AM and always have to have it with a doughnut, try changing to sweetened tea instead and take a short walk or stay in your office. If your kids have to have a snack and you find yourself having one with them, try using raw vegetables and fruit for snacks and preparing it ahead of time. This will encourage good nutrition for everyone. Some children seem to have to have something to eat before bedtime but this is not a good plan to develop. Of course, kids have to grow but you do not, so this is a cruel dish of fate for you. I suggest you try to give them a good supper and maybe a small glass of milk or cup of herbal tea before bed (many herbal teas do not need sweetening and you could join them with the tea.) You could also feed them items you don't care for but they like, or you could let them eat by themselves while you prepare their bath. You should have them scrape off their own dishes and rinse them. *Whatever you do, you should not sit and eat with them.* Just because they are hungry and may need food does not mean you do. Eating calories you don't need, can't use, and won't enjoy is a self-defeating thing to do and very hard to undo.

12. Reduce the number of calories you *routinely* eat everyday by 120. One hundred twenty calories is less than one 12 oz regular coke or beer, less than 11 dorito chips, or 8 french fries or 14 potato chips. It is less than 1 small bag of low-fat potato chips, 1 bagel, 1 cup cake, ½ cup ice cream, 5 large black olives, 2 tablespoons of peanuts, 8 cashews. The point here is that you don't have to cut out

very much to reduce your calorie intake per day by 120. On the other hand, 120 lories per day is 3600 calories in 30 days or one month. Since 3500 calories is one pound, you will have lost one pound. In 12 months or one year, you will have lost 12 pounds. The problem seems to be that people generally do not want to be patient. One pound in a month does not seem like enough so as a consequence, they do nothing. However, losing weight is like eating an elephant. You have to do it one bite at a time. You have to lose weight one pound at a time. Losing weight is also like learning to play the piano. You have to practice a little each day. A little a day is the practical way. It is a basic principle of life.

13. Try some new refreshments. Apple cider vinegar and honey together is rich in vitamins and helps with weight loss. An iced green tea with lime cooler is tasty and healthy and good for weight loss too.

14. Don't look at pictures of food, especially desserts. When you don't have any money, it is a good idea not to go shopping. If you want to lose weight, it is a good idea not to look at yummy pictures of high calorie foods - like foods smothered in cheese, deep fried chicken legs, double fudge chocolate cake and so on. Don't get your saliva glands going. Keep temptations at a minimum.

15. Keep low calorie foods handy. Keep a bunch of raw veggies cleaned and ready to eat in a container in the fridge. Crackers and pretzels are good fillers. A small bowl of cereal with a little milk can be enjoyable.

16. Try some natural powder supplements from health food stores and through the internet. You can get powders that you mix with water that provide multiple greens and fruits that are rich in anti-oxidants and promote good digestion. The IVL brands for example are quite tasty.

Yo...chewing is not an exercise...
running late s not an exercise...
jumping to conclusions is not an exercise...

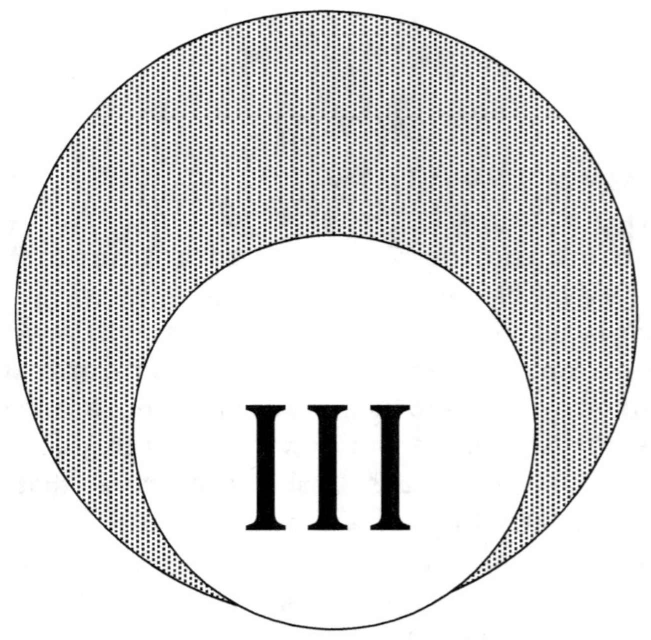

More Thoughts on
Miracles, Myths and Manipulations.

CHAPTER 10

KOOKY DIETS

JUST BECAUSE YOU READ IT IN A MAGAZINE OR BOOK OR SEE IT ON TV OR THE INTERNET DOESN'T MAKE IT TRUE! If you see an article in a newspaper or magazine claiming their product or program can help you lose a lot of weight very quickly - like 5 pounds in 3 days - don't believe it. In one article I saw recently a woman claimed to lose 9 pounds in 4 days. These kinds of articles try to cajole you into buying its product, but its promise is a fantasy, a miracle the size of winning the power ball. Such claims are absolutely irresponsible because real weight loss at that rate simply can't happen. Any average person under any kind of practical and reasonable conditions simply cannot lose 5 pounds in three days. (And even if you could, it is not healthy to lose more than about 2 pounds a week.)

If you use a diuretic and have three to five pounds of water to lose, the scale may show a 5 pound weight loss in three days, but this is not true weight loss. It is also not permanent weight loss. You can bet that this weight will be easily gained back in even a shorter amount of time. Furthermore, after such a weight (water) loss, you could not lose another 5 pounds in the next three days. If this were true weight loss, that should be possible. Just think. Wow, you would lose 20 pounds in less than two weeks!

How do I know this claim is impossible even in the short run? It is a matter of understanding calories in foods and activities, reasonable expectations, and mathematics.

We will assume the most extreme diet, where the *person abstains completely from eating for these three days.* Five pounds is equal to 3500 times 5 or 17,500 calories. Let's suppose the person sleeps 6 hours a night, burning about 60 calories per hour or total of 360 calories per night, or 1080 calories in three nights. Out of the remaining waking time (54 hours) 17,500 - 1080 or 16,420 calories have to be burned off. Then 16,420 calories divided by 54 hours is 304 calories per hour.

This means <u>every</u> waking hour this person has to burn off 304 calories. Let's consider a 140 pound person walking at 3.5 miles/hour. We turn to Table AT140 in the back of this book. Look for the activity "walking at 3.5 mph" and read across to the column headed by 300 (for three hundred calories.) Read the entry 55.6 minutes. This means every hour this person would have to walk 55.6 minutes and then have 4 minutes to rest. Then he/she would have to start walking again. *But remember, no eating.* Mathematically it could be done. But realistically?

Maybe this person could run at 10 mph instead. Find the activity "running 10 mph" and read across to find 18 minutes. This person would have to run 18 minutes out of every hour. Or, if running continuously the person would run 18 minutes x 54 hours or 972 minutes total minutes. Divide by 60 minutes per hour and get 16.2 total hours. To spread it into 3 days, that's 5.4* hours per day. But remember, NO EATING or there will have to be more running because those added calories will have to be burned off too.

I don't know about you, but I find this formidable. Do you know anyone who can run at a 10 mph clip for 5.5 hours straight? We're not talking about athletes and people preparing for marathons. We are talking about ordinary people. We are talking about you. Safer to bet on the horses.

*To be accurate, some calories will be burned off during the approximately 38 hours of non-running (about 12.6 hours a day) so the number of running hours would be slightly less and the 5.4 quoted. But I think - I hope- you get the picture.

A 240 lb person theoretically could work off 564 calories per hour with a 3.5 mph walk. (See table). Again, although the numbers might work, in actuality it is unreasonable to expect a heavily over weight person, to exercise at that level for about 10 hours each day. Discounting people with hard labor jobs, most people cannot do hard activity for 5 or 6 hours a day. People need to set reasonable goals and expectations or they will be discouraged almost right away.

Trying to follow a plan like this is taking the road to failure. The expectation (and promise) is so high that you are doomed before you start. Remember also that losing weight by water loss is lying to yourself. It's a cheat with short benefits. The next morning when you start replenishing your body with the water it craves, you will be devastated when you get on the scales.

We could do a similar analysis on the one suggesting you could lose 9 pounds in 4 days. Suffice it to say, if it is unreasonable to lose 5 pounds in 3 days (equivalent to 1 and 2/3 pounds a day) , then it is unreasonable to lose 9 pounds in 4 days (equivalent to 2 and 1/4 pounds a day.)

Actually, how *reasonable* is it for someone to lose even 1 pound of true weight loss per day only by exercising? We can use Arleen's Tables again to see. First we establish a 24 hour day with 7 hours to sleep, so 17 waking hours. We also establish (generously) that the person will *eat only enough to sustain oneself* so only one pound has to be burned off. One pound is

3500 calories, so divided into 17 hours, that's about 206 calories every hour.

Look at *each* of Arleen's Tables where it says 200 calories at the top and then look for the smallest number in that column. You will find the associated activity in each table is "running at 10 mph." Here are the numbers you should find:

120 pound person - 13.3
140 pound person - 12
160 pound person - 10.8
180 pound person - 9.9
200 pound person - 9.6
220 pound person - 7.2
240 pound person - 7.2

Take these numbers and multiply them by 17 (number of waking hours) to find how many minutes total each pound category person would have to run at 10 mph every day.

The 220 and 240 persons would have to spend 7.2 x 17 = 122.4 minutes running or about 2 total hours every day. The 120 pound person would have spend 13.3 x 17 = 226.1 minutes running or about 3.77 total hours every day.

Because these are the smallest numbers for each person by category in the 200 calorie column, to burn off calories by any other activity would take longer.

So the real question is, is this a reasonable expectation? Is it going to happen? The unhappy conclusion is that it is almost impossible to lose weight by exercise alone. And if you can't lose weight by exercise alone, you will have to, sigh, reduce caloric intake.

Right now advertising on TV there is a diet plan wherein the guy says he lost 20 pounds in 90 days. That's equivalent to 2/9 pounds in 1 day. Somewhere between 1/4 and 1/5 pounds a day and less than 1.5 pounds a week. That's a healthy amount (less than 2 pounds per week), so certainly reasonable! Your next step would be to check to see if you like the plan, the foods, the routine, the price (and any small print.)

Kooky Miracle Soup Diets

There is also a miracle soup diet aka a cabbage soup diet aka wonder soup diet. Soup diets allow you to eat as much of the soup as you want and *guarantee you will lose weight without exercising*. You can even eat the soup between meals.

Soup diets are crash diets and are spectacular in their implied promise. Cabbage soup fans claim you can drop 10 pounds or more in a week (which is either nonsense or extremely risky and unhealthy! Notice they say *can*, not *will*.) However, people do lose weight on them because it's hard to eat more than 1,000 calories a day in soup alone. Soup diets are hard to stick with because they are boring. Some, like the cabbage soup diet, don't supply enough needed nutrients and might leave you feeling weak. *Also, most of the initial weight loss will be due to water loss, not true weight loss.* You'll be hungry a lot too.

Soup diets can guarantee that you will lose some weight without exercising, but the idea that you or anyone can lose 10 pounds in 7 days on this diet is pure nonsense. If you look closer to the claim you will see they carefully inserted the words "up to" before the words "10 pounds". Even with this loop hole keeping it from being a direct lie, the end result is more than just misleading the public. There is also the matter of emotional and psychological damage to all the people who attempt to use this diet and cannot lose what they perceived, the promised (uh, understood) ten pounds.

While you can lose some weight on a soup diet without exercising, here's an easy way to see that you can't lose 10 pounds in 7 days *without exercise*. If you *don't eat anything* for a week, and you burn 2500 calories a day to maintain yourself (I am being generous), then in 7 days you will take in no calories but burn off 2500 x 7 = 17,500 calories. Convert to pounds: divide 17,500 by 3500 and you get (oh rats) 5 pounds! You'll have the strength of jello and the demeanor of a grizzly bear, and you will only be 5 pounds lighter.

If you try this diet and only lose two or three pounds by the end of the week, you will end up thinking that even this diet doesn't work for you. What is wrong with you anyway? Must be your problem is glandular. Woe is you.

On the other hand, they really only promised you could lose *up to* 10 pounds on this diet. If you lose only a *half pound,* that statement is absolutely true — you have lost *up to* 10 pounds. It's a matter of semantics. It's not their problem if you didn't understand what they said.

However, the good news is, the diet *will* work for you. It just won't work at the impossible levels promised. Here is a more reasonable and practical way to use this soup diet. Make up the soup and eat all you want of it one or two days each week — not necessarily and probably better if not two days in a row. You will take in 670 to 804 calories each day you use the "soup plan" (10 to 12 cups of soup per day). Each soup day you would be eating 1300 to 1430 less than what you need, skipping the snacks (using 2100 for your average daily expenditure of energy). In three weeks, eating soup one day a week, you would eat 3900 to 4290 calories less than you need for your average daily expenditure. In three weeks you will lose at least one pound. Not bad.

If you use the soup diet two days a week, you could lose one pound in about ten days or at least two pounds a month. Hey, 2 - 3 pounds a month isn't bad for not having to exercise or starve yourself! That's at least 24 pounds a year!

The danger to using this soup diet (or any diet) the way I have described is that on the non-soup days you may crave to make up for what you couldn't have on the soup days. So you might eat 2 candy bars instead of one, or two doughnuts, or have an extra piece of cake. *The trick is not to change your normal eating routine and diet on the non-soup days.* Otherwise you will take in your usual number of calories per week and wind up losing no weight at all.

Jackie Gleason once designed his own diet plan. He said one week he would eat only hard boiled eggs, and the next week only something else. He pointed out that there are only so many hard boiled eggs you can eat in one week. The problem with such a diet is the unbalanced nutrients. At least with the soup diets, especially if you use the snacks and supplement your diet with vitamins, you will not be putting your body at risk.

Other Miracle Diets

Popping up on facebook and in the news are two new miracle diets. One is Aura Slim Garcinia. Not only can one up lose up to 88 pounds in 60 days, but this new ingredient (from a fruit found only in Asia) kills calories. Really? A calorie is a unit of heat. And there are no "calorie cells". By now you know it is not reasonable to lose even a pound a day. So, you examine the claim from one of the ads:

__Aura Slim Garcinia__ supplement <u>acts as</u> a fat buster, weight buster and appetite suppressant in your body. Performing multiple functions in the body, it <u>can give</u> you a <u>chance to stay slim</u> as well as sexy because of attractive look. It <u>can remove</u> fat stored in different parts of the body; <u>(can) even prevent</u> the further fat to deposit in those areas again.

See, there are no promises. Can act, can remove, can give, can prevent, give a chance. Ha! Now, read the comments by people using it. None report so great results. Some say you have to exercise. Most give no factual results. There is a warning too: <u>Anything less than the correct amount of HCA and dosage will not work effectively.</u> What's the correct amount? Different companies use different amounts. Veer-ry expensive too. (Some cost $100 a bottle.)

Another is the CLA Safflower Oil diet. Have no idea what it's about. But, gotta be good. Khloe Kardashian lost 20 pounds in 20 days! John Goodman lost 67 pounds in 2 months! When you read some of the other comments, those people don't report so much weight loss, and some just say it's wonderful but don't give you any facts. Again, remember losing more than 2 pounds per week is not healthy, and it is not reasonable to lose a pound or more a day.

Pills and Purging

Another type diet plan I would be wary of are the ones that say their pill or drink will raise your metabolism and therefore make you burn calories faster. I would not advise anyone to play around with their body chemistry without having the supervision of a legitimate doctor. The body can tolerate a lot of abuse, but my instinct tells me this is either a scam or might potentially affect your health.

Then there is bulimia. Bulimia involves a cycle of binging and purging. Bulimia may seem to work at first but ultimately affects your teeth, mouth, esophagus, stomach, heart. It negatively affects many organs in the body, and can cause serious medical complications. If you can't lose weight using a structured legitimate diet or disciplined weight management, you should work with a doctor and nutritionist. Bulimia is very dangerous.

Conclusions

There's a moral to all this, as you would expect. The moral is: When you try to lose five pounds in three days, -- or nine pounds in four days -- or 10 pounds in a week -- you will not only **not** lose that weight, *but you will convince yourself that you cannot lose weight.* Losing weight is just too difficult if not impossible. Yes, you are right. Losing weight *is* too difficult approached this way.

The truth is, if you really want to lose weight, stay away from quick fixes and miracle cures. Don't believe everything you read. You can't hurry weight loss. As I said before, you didn't wake up one morning and find yourself 10 or 20 pounds overweight. You will certainly not get skinny overnight either. You are simply going to have to commit yourself to two things:

1. a change of eating habits from ground up (not just what you eat but how you eat)

2. PATIENCE.

This might be an unpleasant fact. You may wish you never read this. You may feel like throwing this book out right now. (If you do, rip it in two first and give it several good heaves so that you burn up a few calories doing it. Don't just drop it gently in the waste basket.)

However, if what I said is not true, then why are so many people on yo-yo diets, or diets that work only while they are "on them"? Why do so many people claim that they cannot lose weight? A really good diet plan can work wonders to get you started, but if you do not learn to change your eating and social habits while you are using the diet plan, then nothing that is important in weight management really changes and becomes part of you. You didn't learn anything. You are stuck with the same old you once you are "off" the diet. Therefore, you can plan on gaining that weight back shortly thereafter because you are going to revert to the same eating and social habits that you were using when you gained that weight in the first place. And if this is going to be the case, why bother submitting yourself to all that effort and all that pain?

I wish I was as fat
as I was the first time
I thought I was fat.

Chapter 11

Myths, Mistakes, Lies, Rationalizations

1. You can't go wrong with yogurt.

Sort of. If it doesn't have over 20 grams of sugar and if there is no high fructose in it. The best yogurts have probiotics.

2. High fructose corn syrup (HFCS) is not that bad.

Major, major misconception. HFCS is made from corn sugar, not cane sugar. Cane and corn sugar are not the same and are digested differently. Products with HFCS are sweeter and cheaper and if on the label is a marker for poor-quality, nutritionally-depleted, processed food. When HFCS is used in moderation it is a major cause of heart disease, obesity, cancer, dementia, liver failure, tooth decay, and more. The average American increased their consumption of HFCS (mostly from sugar sweetened drinks and processed food) from zero to over 60 pounds per person per year. During that time period, obesity rates more than tripled and diabetes incidence increased more than seven fold. Not perhaps the only cause, but a fact that cannot be ignored. (Look at the research available on the internet. The article by Mark Hyman MD is especially clear and straight forward.) *High fructose corn syrup (HFCS) is definitely not good for your body.*

3. Cereal Bars are OK.

Maybe. You'll need to do a comprehensive search to make sure they do not contain corn syrup HFCS. Some bars contain sugar and corn syrup both. I'm not saying no to cereal bars. I'm saying be careful. This is a warning. They may also have more calories that you expect.

4. It makes a difference what you eat when you are dieting.

Wrong. Nutrition wise there is a difference in diets and certainly you want to make sure you are getting enough nutrients. But energy wise, the body can't tell the difference between fried chicken, ice cream or raw carrot sticks. As soon as you eat more raw carrot sticks above what you burn off, you will gain weight.

5. Sugar free, sugarless, and diabetic labels on a serving means less calories in that serving.

Not necessarily. To make up for flavor lost, fats and other ingredients are added, and some will increase the number of calories.

6. One should purchase low calorie and reduced calories items.

Also not necessarily. By definition and law, low calorie foods may not have more than 40 calories in a portion, and reduced calorie items have to have 1/3 less calories per portion. However, they may have made their portions really small. <u>Your</u> usual portion may have more calories than they led you to believe.

A. Watkins

7. Fasting one or two days a week would work.

Not advisable. Fasting is fairly ineffective. Fasting (limiting food intake to all but water) will cause the body to lose muscle as well as fat. Then the metabolic rate decreases and the body burns fewer calories. Losing weight becomes much harder. Besides that, the person will often take in too much food when the fast is over, and the excess will turn into fat rather than muscle.

8. We can only buy a big serving so we have to eat it.

Why? Eat what you want and toss the rest. It's called "eat and heave."

9. Overweight people have a predisposition to be fat and when they try to lose weight, this causes problems with their health.

Putting aside that some people may have a real glandular problem that causes them to be fat, and some people may be taking drugs which cause them to gain weight, this is most likely a rationalization. There may be some people who should work with a psychologist to deal with ingrained habits. Most people, however, are overweight because they eat too much.

10. People get fat from eating fat.

People get fat from eating more calories than they burn off. It makes no difference where the calories come from. In fact, a favored diet is the Atkins diet. On that plan people eat more fat and eat very little carbohydrates. People like this diet because people like the flavor of various fats in foods, and fat makes people feel more full. Despite the fat, the plan has people eat fewer calories than they burn so they lose weight.

11. Exercise is over-rated for shedding pounds.

True. Most studies find that people lose more weight when they're told to cut calories rather than to exercise more. "People totally overestimate how many calories they'll burn when they exercise," explains Roberts, director of the Energy Metabolism Laboratory at Tufts University in Boston. Roberts says individual responses to a controlled exercise program showed huge variability. Those who lost the least weight also reported more hunger and ate more on a given day near the end of the study than did those who lost the most weight.

12. Muscles help burn calories

"Muscle is more metabolically active than fat," says Roberts. "So if you have five more pounds of muscle and five pounds less fat, it will make a bit of difference, but not a huge difference. Weight control is dominated by how many calories you eat. That's the honest truth." Don't count on exercise alone to lose or keep off extra pounds.

13. You can speed up your metabolism.

"This boosting of metabolism is pretty overblown," Roberts says. "Magazines and supplements love to talk about ways to boost your metabolism. But you can eat a brownie with 700 calories in about 10 seconds, and there is nothing that you can remotely do to change your metabolism by anywhere near that much, except maybe to give up your job and spend all your time in the gym." Don't expect to lose much weight from "metabolism boosters."

A. Watkins

14. Portion and Serving sizes are the same.

Not necessarily. A *portion* is how much food you choose to eat at one time. A serving size is the amount of food listed (and recommended) in the Dietary Guidelines* for Americans. Sometimes, the portion size and serving size match; sometimes they don't. A serving is a standard amount used to help give advice about how much to eat, or to identify how many calories and nutrients are in a food. When eating, it's the size of your portions that really count!

15. Misinformation can lead to weight gain.

Yes. If you continually underestimate the amount of calories you eat in an item or by day, overestimate the recommended portion sizes, and overestimate the number of calories lost by exercise, you can't win the fat war. If you weigh more than you should, consider if you have faulty thoughts in any of these three areas. Remember in one way or another, you are responsible for every calorie.

Dear Diet,
Things are just not going to work out between us. It's not me, it's you. You are tasteless and boring, and I can't stop cheating on you.

Chapter 12

Your Body as a Machine!

The things I have been telling you have mostly to do with maintaining your weight or losing just a little. However, I do have things to say about the way you might want to diet and the things you might want to put into our body. I start with an analogy.

If you put inferior low grade fuel into your new car, it might ping or not climb that hill efficiently. Maybe it will deposit soot and carbon in various unwanted places, cause a loud muffler. If you do not keep the car well supplied with the correct oil, the motor will get gunked up and eventually stop. If you don't clean the windows or light shields, you will have trouble seeing. If you use the brakes too hard, they will wear thin faster. And if you do not fix your brakes when they are thin, you may find they squeal or won't stop you in time. You need the proper amount of air in the tires, the right transmission oil. You may even get annoying rattles and doors that stick, electric windows that don't open. There are many things that you need to do to make your car operate at top efficiency.

Your body works like a machine too. Your body *is* a physical and chemical machine. The way the body conducts its business - digesting food, converting food into energy, discarding what it can't use - can be analogous to your car. You need to have nutritional foods which come from a balanced diet of protein, carbohydrates and fats. The more you give the body what it needs and wants, the better your body will work for a longer time. The less you put into your body that takes the place of something it needs, the less it has to work with to stay healthy.

Your body is at least as smart as a car. It knows what it needs and tries to tell you. I believe it wants real butter, real milk, real sugar, real meat. Not a lot, but some. If you give your body man made oils, cream, sweeteners it will be like making your body tread water. For example, items made with high fructose are incredibly sweet and high in calories. Yet your body will still want plain old sugar in the short run. But worse, in the long run, your body may get used to that sweetness, and one thing for sure, your taste buds will come to want that sweetness which is different from sugar sweetness. The more your body can't use what you put into it even though it has a caloric value, the more it is going to nag you into eating, hoping you will finally pick something to eat that it needs.

I believe you can become somewhat addicted to these false or empty "nutrients". Whether or not that is true, it is true that the body suffers when it doesn't get sufficient amounts of all the nutrients it needs to build and repair cells and regulate the various bodily processes.

Then there are the additives. For flavor, for color, for keeping the ice cream from running, to keep foods fresh, to keep substances mixed and uniformed, enhance texture, protect foods from drying out, keep powdered foods flowing. There's also what may be still on the food, like pesticides and fertilizers. To eat foods enhanced, or infused with preservatives, food coloring, gum additives, etc, which makes them softer, spread easier, stay softer, stay dry or stay crunchy, stay "unstuck", be less runny, have good texture, - is in my opinion to abuse the body. Your body must try to do things it wasn't designed to do or make do with what it gets.

The only reason your body doesn't break down immediately when you mistreat it, is because your body tolerates a lot of nutritional insults. The body adjusts within reason to the things we do and eat. It overlooks and excuses a wide range of dietary and physical behaviors that are far from ideal. Of course it will not tolerate blatant abuse forever.

Here is another factor about weight gain and a healthy body to consider. The more you put into your body over what it really needs to function properly, the more your body has to store that somewhere if it can't wash it out. It may store it as fat which you see, or it may store it in the kidneys or corrode your heart valves, or cause you gout or diabetes or a form of heart disease.

The primary purpose of eating is to supply our body with the ingredients (nutrients, proteins, carbohydrates etc.) it needs to run efficiently. However, our love affair with food seems to have nothing to do with that. It would almost seem, when one looks at what people eat, that the principle reasons we eat are taste and comfort. We like to chew and taste and put things in our mouths. We like to sit with other people and socialize over food. We like to smell it and look at it, see it molded and shaped, creamed and displayed like an art. If this were not so, we would buy pills that would give us precisely what we needed and go on with our other interests.

I believe the more things we eat that are natural, the more likely we will feel satisfied and the more likely it is that we will be eating healthy foods, foods which contain the nutrients that our bodies need and crave.

As an end note, let me be clear that we do not have to walk the fine line nutritionists seem to be telling us. If this were not so, we would have more clear, definitive outcomes regarding weight research and more immediate, devastating perhaps, responses to changes in our diets.

You should eat the best food per calorie you can afford to eat on your calorie budget, and not the poorest nutritionally. From the best foods you will get the most satisfaction, the best energy, the best health, and the enjoyment of knowing it is the best without having to feel guilty about it. Don't eat what you do not want because it is cheap. It is worth the cost to buy good nutritional food when paying the price of eating poorly is expensive to your health.

Eat less and exercise more?
That's the most ridiculous fad diet I
ever heard of.

I feel like I've been on a diet for 3 months but it's only been since 9 am.

Chapter 13

Let Science, Technology, Somebody Else Do It

We want science and technology to do the hard work for us. We want it to help us grow hair, lower cholesterol, lose weight, lower blood pressure, grow taller, make us potent, get rid of acne, have larger breasts, and things like that in addition to keeping us well. This despite the fact that many of these things are either controllable by diet and exercise, or are cosmetic and unnecessary. Most of us would rather take a pill than raise our little finger to help ourselves.

Money and time are required to develop a new medication or medical product like artificial hearts, knees, hips, ear implants and so forth. Untold numbers have been relieved of pain or even regained their lives because of research and technology. Much more can be done. It takes a lot of time and effort and creativity to develop a medication or product to the point where the FDA will allow it to be released for public use. Even then, they and insurance companies plant a watchful eye on them.

During the development phase, in addition to testing and retesting, there are other impediments to bringing the product onto the market. One is that people don't want to have any side effects or failures. If anything goes wrong – even if we don't need that operation and are told up front that it is not always successful, or that something may go bad with some people – if anything goes wrong, we want the right to sue. The sad end result of this is that sometimes products have been taken off the market when for most people they have been very effective. Other products have not been fully developed because of cost and fear of litigation.

Whether the product is medicinal or cosmetic, after all the preliminaries, sometimes the research has to be continued on animals. Generally people do not want animal experiments and they should be avoided if there is another way. But sometimes a life saving drug is developed that we would know nothing about if it weren't for experimenting first on animals.

We live in a world where things have become so very complicated and convoluted and the public is so poorly educated in logic, history, science, mathematics and so on, that people naively expect the impossible to be accomplished by immaculate conception. It appears that many people have become capable of believing anything and expecting everything. Facts are on an even keel with lies because people can't tell the difference, and wouldn't know how to go about finding out which is which if they did. Just as our society no longer is one where moral persuasion and ostracism directs people to modify and control their behavior, but use the law to force people to do what is perceived correct or suitable, the same way people no longer care to be in control of their bodies and thoughts but prefer some quick fix like a weight loss pill or some anti-depressant drug. The locus of control is no longer within, where one's abilities, talents, and brains are. When the locus of control is outside the person, therein comes the blaming someone else, holding something else responsible, pointing to our skin color, our unchangeable past, our height, our divorced parents whatever seems appropriate at the time.

Always looking for an easy way to do the disliked thing, all kinds of fads seduce us into emptying our pockets in the hope we will be thinner, less wrinkled, grow more hair, have nicer skin, better sex drive. One need only go into the drug store and walk through the cosmetic section to see the vast variety of ingredients promising to do the same thing. How can one chose? What should one believe? Can they all be right? Can they all be wrong? How did they decide what to put in their product to accomplish their claim?

The way to challenge these claims for ourselves is to take a common sense approach. For example, people have been eating all kinds of foods for centuries. Animal fats, natural butter, fruit off the vine, eggs, coffee etc. No one seems to be dying of caffeine or sugar or eggs or even potato chips from what I read in the papers. Perhaps they do when they eat too much of these foods over a long period of time or in some combination that we don't know about – but is that a reason to eliminate these foods or feel guilty about eating them?

It is unlikely that our ancestors ate gobs of these foods because they just weren't available. So maybe we should just moderate the amounts we eat. And in the same vein, they weren't eating all those additives, all that fake, junk stuff.

Big food companies make lots of money off their products. They want to keep it that way. They see people are working and are busy. Kids are flying everywhere, there's another birthday party, mom can't walk very good, dad is losing his mental abilities (and you are losing your mind.) So where's that food I can stick in the microwave or add hot water to? Where's something easy the kids can heat up. Where's that stuff I can buy 10 pounds of and it will keep forever? That milk that won't go sour, the ice cream that won't melt, that bread that won't get stale or moldy?

Cheese. Let's put cheese on everything so even Styrofoam will taste good. Can you heat it right in the box? Wonderful! It's all passed by the FDA. This means you will not die from it - today. No promises about long term results. Accumulate in the body? Interact with other additives, with the meds you are taking? Make your body work too hard to flush it out? Not known. Don't think about it.

This is a good time to talk again about high glucose syrup. This stuff is sweeter than natural sugar. And it is practically everywhere except cigarettes. Pick up a can of spaghetti sauce? Why does spaghetti sauce have to be sweet? If word gets out it is not good for you or pays off in a lot of calories, then they can change it a bit, whatever they have to do, and call it another name. It is usually a glucose name though. People get used to that sweet taste and after awhile it becomes almost an addiction. If it is not in the food, the food doesn't taste right. We got stuck to it. If you want to get away from that, you need to start cooking yourself.

Unfortunately, we *want* the food companies to do what they are doing. We want to have our lives, and we need somebody to help us. We don't have nannies, or extended families anymore. Only rich people have cooks.

Furthermore, food companies are making us think serving sizes are bigger than they are. In most drinks there are 2 servings. Check it out. Also, look at those small bags of chips. How many servings? Most are 2.5 servings. I looked at some banana chips. Says 110 calories. BUT that's for ONE serving, about 8 chips! Here's another. Cheddar sour cream potato chips. 160 calories in a serving. How many chips in a serving? About 11. You were planning to eat the whole bag full, weren't you? You can do the math. In both cases, about 14 calories per chip. Eat the whole bag of sour cream chips and diminish your calorie bank by 400 calories. Eating chips and drinking pop will suck your calorie bank dry in a jiffy.

Unfortunately, you can't get through the day without being faced with food at least three times, to say nothing about when you want a snack. Then there's the phone calls or visits from friends. Or maybe your kid wants a cookie. Or you go shopping. There they are, those hotdog/ pepsi carts or the delis in the big markets so you never have to be hungry.

Why, all of life is against you, all of society. All the big guys that want to sell you food, clothes, diet plans, books, exercise equipment. They are all against you. If they were on your side they would hang a bag of potato chips on the rack with the bikinis, and put scales in front of ice cream stations. Every food item would be marked clearly with a warning: You will have to run for 10 minutes to work off the calories in this cookie – which will cost you 89 cents.

They like you spending money for a new diet plan, book or exercise machine. Also, you can buy some of those really tight elastic clothes that pull your body in and make it seem as tight and solid as it should be without manufactured help (and in which you feel like a stuffed sausage). Don't ever think to ask yourself if all that squeezing of your body is good for you. Because if it isn't somebody will come out with something else that will cover up the broken veins or some new program to condition you up (providing you buy it and use it.) More work! More money!

Nutrition Science is always evolving. In the 80's, fats were bad. People listened and turned to pastas and bagels and fat free cookies. Then we were told it was OK to eat *good* fats, so we started using olive oil and eating almonds. Restaurants served us specialty breads to dip in oil and vinegar and put avocado slices on our burgers. Then we were told to ration our intake of eggs and not eat an egg breakfast every day despite the fact that farmers had been doing that for umpteen years.

Then we found out that eggs with its cholesterol not only wasn't so bad, but that the body itself makes cholesterol. Then came the good and bad cholesterol. Today the emphasis is on overall eating patterns. In other words, it's not about eggs, it's about eggs and everything we eat with them. It's about the whole eating profile, not about individual foods. We should stop using diets that target individual foods to either eat or shun and start looking at eating patterns. In other words, as I have been saying, eat what you like and want, just don't overdo it. A healthy dietary pattern is far superior to can/can't eat diets. And you won't have to upgrade to the next fad diet that comes along which also won't work in the long run.

If you are on one of those good food/bad food diets where you have to eat something you do not like or can't eat something you really like in order to lose weight and you know you are not going to eat that way when you are at your goal weight, then that is not a proper diet for you. You need to choose a diet that you can stick with, well yes…, forever. You will not be happy if you can't eat certain foods that you like. The truth of the matter is, you do not need a diet plan at all. You need a weight management plan.

People who overeat need to find ways to change their eating habits so that eating is still a satisfying experience. Diets present emotional conflicts between desiring food, and then denying it or feeling guilty about eating it. The bottom line for everyone is to understand the rules and self-discipline.

No matter what society tells you or how many books you read, no matter what technology and pharmaceuticals are available, there is only one truism: If you take in more calories than you burn off, you will gain weight; If you take in less calories than you burn off you will lose weight.

The government will never provide a program which will operate in opposition to this. No law can ever be passed to change it. Popular opinion to the contrary will never prevail, and wishful thinking will never win. You might as well accept the fact right now that this is something you will have to do yourself. And you will do it only through self-discipline and patience.

The only thing diets and/or other people can do is give you a menu which guarantees you will take in fewer calories than you burn and still be nutritional if you follow it. It doesn't really matter which one you choose, so choose one you like. Or not. Or just use methods suggested in this book to manage your weight. *If you can change the way you think about eating, you can change your eating habits and you can think your way to a slimmer, healthier body. Be patient and a believer, and you will be happier.*

What about those diets that are built around things like gluten-free, low-glycemic index, high- protein, low- carb, antioxidant-rich, paleo and probiotic diets, to name some? Does it sound complicated? Does it put you off? Make you feel doomed before you start? The answer is simple. You do not need to know all this stuff about fats and sugars and transfats and additives to lose weight. All you need to know is 3500 calories is worth one pound.

I think a dieter should not have to look at a list of things that tell him or her what they can eat and what they can't and how much. I think a dieter should not have to enter into a new world of strange and unappetizing foods like someone being transported into outer space. I think a dieter should feel like he or she is still in the same world and just as normal as normal can be. I think a dieter should not have to tell everyone they are on a diet like they have some disease and are on some drug to get cured. I think a dieter should not have to do crazy math or learn some complicated "point system", or measure out or weigh their food. And they certainly should not have to isolate themselves from the world to succeed.

In regular dieting, people make excuses for volunteering to get off the wagon whenever it seems appropriate. A special get together (birthday, graduation, memorial, reunion, etc), a smorgasbord, potluck, holiday party etc. While this isn't viewed as *voluntary backsliding*, it is, and the damage to the overall diet can be devastating to the goal of losing any significant amount of weight. With a weight management diet, you do not have to worry about backsliding. You are constantly eating anything you want in a limited amount. Like that yummy double quarter pounder with cheese you can't resist. You can eat half today and half tomorrow. Similarly, you do not have to eat two pieces of pie today and a supersized cheeseburger because you are not going to be allowed to eat that tomorrow or the next day.

When you are trying to lose weight, any day you eat less than you burn off is a good day. But when you eat those "saved" calories and sometimes more the next day, you have shot yourself in the foot. In weight management you prevent those irresistible cravings. You know you can have some tomorrow. In weight management also you work with the whole picture, the whole week so to speak, not hour by hour. Like driving around potholes. You don't go exactly straight and you see where you are going better by looking ahead and not at each pothole.

If you have decided to work with a good planned diet and you backslide, do not be so discouraged thinking you have blown your diet that you give up and eat gobs of other things you were not supposed to eat. That's like losing a dollar bill and then opening your wallet and dumping out the rest of your cash. Or making a wrong turn so going on to Phoenix instead of Benson. No one eats a piece of cheese cake or pizza and wakes up a pound heavier. Forget it. After a half dozen or so of these relapses, you will wind up losing a little less over the year than you planned. Still good.

Here is a *thinking caution* though: Our bodies in an odd way seem to like to stay at the weight we are at, whether we want to lose weight or gain weight. It seems to me from personal experience that you have to fight to lose that first several pounds. Then after it realizes you are not going to be giving it as many calories each day that it was used to, it adjusts to the new weight. Weight loss (or gain) seems to go through a stepping process rather than flow smoothly. I think this is why sometimes it seems you can eat 3 extra pieces of pie and not gain any weight and sometimes you practically fast for three days and don't lose any.

Weight loss seems to hit plateaus during which you get frustrated and start to think you aren't losing weight anymore. During these times you are truly tempted to throw in the towel and give up. However, this is when you have to have faith that eating fewer calories than you need to maintain your basic needs is still working. You have to reach inside yourself and pull out all the strength you have to stay focused on your goal. You have to believe what you are doing is going to pay off.

I named my dog five miles
so I could say I walk five miles every day.

only one calorie per serving,
a million servings per can.

Chapter 14

If You Want to Lose More Weight Faster

This book is written primarily to help people lose a little weight and to maintain their weight. I do not have any diet program to recommend. Pick any diet program you like and think you can stick with. All these *legitimate* diets will provide you ways to cut back calories and you will lose weight on all of them *provided you follow them.*

Having written that, if **I** were seriously trying to lose a lot of weight, 20-30 or more pounds, here is what **I** would do:

I would get on the internet and look for low calorie recipes. There has to be hundreds if not thousands on there. I would make up my own recipe book and put in there everything I thought I would really like along with the calorie count. I'd aim for 100 or more recipes of 300 - 600 calories. Then I would make one of these meals every day according to my taste mood, and prepare them for the meal when I usually eat the most. I wouldn't let myself be hungry. I would, however, let myself eat something I really craved. So to start, the only change I would make would be the replacement of that one meal. (*This also means I would not eat an extra doughnut at breakfast or an extra anything anytime. If you want to lose weight, you can't cheat.*)

I would understand that when I go on somebody else's diet plan, no matter how they do it, all they are going to do is restrict the number of calories I eat. I would understand that I was giving them the power to tell me what to eat and when and how often. Besides that, I'd know how guilty I would feel whenever I messed up.

On the other hand, I would know I could design my own low calorie diet plan with good nutritional meals using recipes I liked from the internet. These would be meals I liked and could use for the rest of my life, if I wanted to. I wouldn't have to pay anybody for something that should be easy enough to do by myself with the help of the internet. I might not even like what they wanted me to eat anyway.

Look, it's hard to follow a diet somebody makes for you, even if they give you some leeway and some variety. When you choose your own recipes it's not like a real diet because you are making the choices, choices you want to make. You've made a commitment to yourself. Also meals won't be boring because you will have lots of recipes. When - yes when - you start to lose weight, then you might think about eating fewer calories at other meals because you will feel encouraged.

The one other thing I would do is walk one mile every day. That would increase my energy expenditure a little, and walking is so very good for the body. When you are walking, think about what a blessing it is to be able to walk. Think of all the people who can't walk because of some disease or physical problem. Think of those in their upper years who can't walk because they are too overweight. Think of you in your later years ahead. Promise yourself that won't be you.

Remember, weight loss (or gain) seems to go through a stepping process rather than flow smoothly, hitting plateaus during which it is easy to get frustrated. But don't give up.

A. Watkins

Eating fewer calories than you need to maintain your basic needs is still working. What you are doing is going to pay off.

I've added a few minutes to that hour glass figure
I had I high school.

the box said it was two pounds of chocolate,
so why did I gain 10 pounds?

Arleen's Tables

Tables for Weights 120 - 240 Pounds

DIRECTIONS

1. Determine the number of calories in the article of food you want to eat.

2. Identify the activity (row) you want to use to burn off those calories.

3. Find the column heading that is closest to the number of calories in your food item. (You may have to add two column headings to get the closest amount.)

4. Find the corresponding number of minutes in the row by column entry. If you use two columns, find both numbers and add them.

AT120

120 pound person

***Number of minutes needed to burn off calories
given in 10 calorie intervals***

cal/min	calorie intervals	10 min	20 min	30 min	40 min	50 min
	activities					
3.8	aquaerobics	2.6	5.3	7.9	10.5	13.2
7.4	aerobics, medium	1.4	2.7	4.1	5.4	6.8
4.7	walking 3.5 mph	2.1	4.3	6.4	8.5	10.6
9.4	jogging (6.5 mph)	1.1	2.1	3.2	4.3	5.3
15	running (10 mph)	0.7	1.3	2.0	2.7	3.3
3.6	cycling (5.5 mph)	2.8	5.6	8.3	11.1	13.9
7.7	soccer	1.3	2.6	3.9	5.2	6.5
8.2	raquetball	1.2	2.4	3.7	4.9	6.1
6	tennis- rec	1.7	3.3	5.0	6.7	8.3
3.8	ping pong	2.6	5.3	7.9	10.5	13.2
9.4	martial arts	1.1	2.1	3.2	4.3	5.3
7	swimming laps	1.4	2.9	4.3	5.7	7.1
4.6	golf -carry clubs	2.2	4.3	6.5	8.7	10.9
3.3	pilates	3.0	6.1	9.1	12.1	15.2
2.4	yoga	4.2	8.3	12.5	16.7	20.8
1.4	driving car	7.1	14.3	21.4	28.6	35.7
1.2	lying or sitting	8.3	16.7	25.0	33.3	41.7
1.5	standing quietly	6.7	13.3	20.0	26.7	33.3
1.5	computer work	6.7	13.3	20.0	26.7	33.3

AT120(cont)

120 pound person

**Number of minutes needed to burn off calories
given in 10 calorie intervals**

60	70	80	90	100	200	300	400
min	min	min	min	min	min	min	min
15.8	18.4	21.1	23.7	26.3	52.6	78.9	105.3
8.1	9.5	10.8	12.2	13.5	27.0	40.5	54.1
12.8	14.9	17.0	19.1	21.3	42.6	63.8	85.1
6.4	7.4	8.5	9.6	10.6	21.3	31.9	42.6
4.0	4.7	5.3	6.0	6.7	13.3	20.0	26.7
16.7	19.4	22.2	25.0	27.8	55.6	83.3	111.1
7.8	9.1	10.4	11.7	13.0	26.0	39.0	51.9
7.3	8.5	9.8	11.0	12.2	24.4	36.6	48.8
10.0	11.7	13.3	15.0	16.7	33.3	50.0	66.7
15.8	18.4	21.1	23.7	26.3	52.6	78.9	105.3
6.4	7.4	8.5	9.6	10.6	21.3	31.9	42.6
8.6	10.0	11.4	12.9	14.3	28.6	42.9	57.1
13.0	15.2	17.4	19.6	21.7	43.5	65.2	87.0
18.2	21.2	24.2	27.3	30.3	60.6	90.9	121.2
25.0	29.2	33.3	37.5	41.7	83.3	125.0	166.7
42.9	50.0	57.1	64.3	71.4	142.9	214.3	285.7
50.0	58.3	66.7	75.0	83.3	166.7	250.0	333.3
40.0	46.7	53.3	60.0	66.7	133.3	200.0	266.7
40.0	46.7	53.3	60.0	66.7	133.3	200.0	266.7

AT140

140 pound person
Number of minutes needed to burn off calories
given in 10 calorie intervals

	calorie intervals	10	20	30	40	50
		min	min	min	min	min
cal/min	activities					
4.4	aquaerobics	2.3	4.5	6.8	9.1	11.4
6.4	aerobics, medium	1.6	3.1	4.7	6.3	7.8
5.4	walking 3.5 mph	1.9	3.7	5.6	7.4	9.3
11.1	jogging (6.5 mph)	0.9	1.8	2.7	3.6	4.5
16.7	running (10 mph)	0.6	1.2	1.8	2.4	3.0
4.2	cycling (5.5 mph)	2.4	4.8	7.1	9.5	11.9
8.5	soccer	1.2	2.4	3.5	4.7	5.9
9.4	raquetball	1.1	2.1	3.2	4.3	5.3
6.8	tennis- recreational	1.5	2.9	4.4	5.9	7.4
4.2	ping pong	2.4	4.8	7.1	9.5	11.9
11.1	martial arts	0.9	1.8	2.7	3.6	4.5
8.2	swimming laps	1.2	2.4	3.7	4.9	6.1
5.4	golf (pull, carry clubs)	1.9	3.7	5.6	7.4	9.3
3.9	pilates	2.6	5.1	7.7	10.3	12.8
2.8	yoga	3.6	7.1	10.7	14.3	17.9
1.5	driving car	6.7	13.3	20.0	26.7	33.3
1.4	lying or sitting quietly	7.1	14.3	21.4	28.6	35.7
1.7	standing quietly	5.9	11.8	17.6	23.5	29.4
1.7	typing on cumputer	5.9	11.8	17.6	23.5	29.4

AT140(cont)

140 pound person

Number of minutes needed to burn off calories given in 10 calorie intervals

60	70	80	90	100	200	300	400
min	min	min	min	min	min	min	min
13.6	15.9	18.2	20.5	22.7	45.5	68.2	90.9
9.4	10.9	12.5	14.1	15.6	31.3	46.9	62.5
11.1	13.0	14.8	16.7	18.5	37.0	55.6	74.1
5.4	6.3	7.2	8.1	9.0	18.0	27.0	36.0
3.6	4.2	4.8	5.4	6.0	12.0	18.0	24.0
14.3	16.7	19.0	21.4	23.8	47.6	71.4	95.2
7.1	8.2	9.4	10.6	11.8	23.5	35.3	47.1
6.4	7.4	8.5	9.6	10.6	21.3	31.9	42.6
8.8	10.3	11.8	13.2	14.7	29.4	44.1	58.8
14.3	16.7	19.0	21.4	23.8	47.6	71.4	95.2
5.4	6.3	7.2	8.1	9.0	18.0	27.0	36.0
7.3	8.5	9.8	11.0	12.2	24.4	36.6	48.8
11.1	13.0	14.8	16.7	18.5	37.0	55.6	74.1
15.4	17.9	20.5	23.1	25.6	51.3	76.9	102.6
21.4	25.0	28.6	32.1	35.7	71.4	107.1	142.9
40.0	46.7	53.3	60.0	66.7	133.3	200.0	266.7
42.9	50.0	57.1	64.3	71.4	142.9	214.3	285.7
35.3	41.2	47.1	52.9	58.8	117.6	176.5	235.3
35.3	41.2	47.1	52.9	58.8	117.6	176.5	235.3

AT160

160 pound person
Number of minutes needed to burn off calories given in 10 calorie intervals

	calorie intervals	10 min	20 min	30 min	40 min	50 min
cal/min	activities					
5.1	aquaerobics	2.0	3.9	5.9	7.8	9.8
7.3	aerobics, medium	1.4	2.7	4.1	5.5	6.8
6.3	walking 3.5 mph	1.6	3.2	4.8	6.3	7.9
12.5	jogging (6.5 mph)	0.8	1.6	2.4	3.2	4.0
18.5	running (10 mph)	0.5	1.1	1.6	2.2	2.7
4.7	cycling (5.5 mph)	2.1	4.3	6.4	8.5	10.6
9.8	soccer	1.0	2.0	3.1	4.1	5.1
10.8	raquetball	0.9	1.9	2.8	3.7	4.6
7.7	tennis- recreational	1.3	2.6	3.9	5.2	6.5
4.8	ping pong	2.1	4.2	6.3	8.3	10.4
12.8	martial arts	0.8	1.6	2.3	3.1	3.9
9.4	swimming laps	1.1	2.1	3.2	4.3	5.3
6.2	golf (pull, carry clubs)	1.6	3.2	4.8	6.5	8.1
4.4	pilates	2.3	4.5	6.8	9.1	11.4
3.2	yoga	3.1	6.3	9.4	12.5	15.6
1.6	driving car	6.3	12.5	18.8	25.0	31.3
1.5	lying or sitting quietly	6.7	13.3	20.0	26.7	33.3
1.9	standing quietly	5.3	10.5	15.8	21.1	26.3
1.9	typing on cumputer	5.3	10.5	15.8	21.1	26.3

AT160(cont)

160 pound person

*Number of minutes needed to burn off calories
given in 10 calorie intervals*

60	70	80	90	100	200	300	400
min	min	min	min	min	min	min	min
11.8	13.7	15.7	17.6	19.6	39.2	58.8	78.4
8.2	9.6	11.0	12.3	13.7	27.4	41.1	54.8
9.5	11.1	12.7	14.3	15.9	31.7	47.6	63.5
4.8	5.6	6.4	7.2	8.0	16.0	24.0	32.0
3.2	3.8	4.3	4.9	5.4	10.8	16.2	21.6
12.8	14.9	17.0	19.1	21.3	42.6	63.8	85.1
6.1	7.1	8.2	9.2	10.2	20.4	30.6	40.8
5.6	6.5	7.4	8.3	9.3	18.5	27.8	37.0
7.8	9.1	10.4	11.7	13.0	26.0	39.0	51.9
12.5	14.6	16.7	18.8	20.8	41.7	62.5	83.3
4.7	5.5	6.3	7.0	7.8	15.6	23.4	31.3
6.4	7.4	8.5	9.6	10.6	21.3	31.9	42.6
9.7	11.3	12.9	14.5	16.1	32.3	48.4	64.5
13.6	15.9	18.2	20.5	22.7	45.5	68.2	90.9
18.8	21.9	25.0	28.1	31.3	62.5	93.8	125.0
37.5	43.8	50.0	56.3	62.5	125.0	187.5	250.0
40.0	46.7	53.3	60.0	66.7	133.3	200.0	266.7
31.6	36.8	42.1	47.4	52.6	105.3	157.9	210.5
31.6	36.8	42.1	47.4	52.6	105.3	157.9	210.5

AT180

180 pound person
Number of minutes needed to burn off calories
given in 10 calorie intervals

	calorie intervals	10	20	30	40	50
		min	min	min	min	min
cal/min	activities					
5.7	aquaerobics	1.8	3.5	5.3	7.0	8.8
8.2	aerobics, medium	1.2	2.4	3.7	4.9	6.1
7	walking 3.5 mph	1.4	2.9	4.3	5.7	7.1
14.3	jogging (6.5 mph)	0.7	1.4	2.1	2.8	3.5
20.2	running (10 mph)	0.5	1.0	1.5	2.0	2.5
5.3	cycling (5.5 mph)	1.9	3.8	5.7	7.5	9.4
10.9	soccer	0.9	1.8	2.8	3.7	4.6
12.2	raquetball	0.8	1.6	2.5	3.3	4.1
8.7	tennis- recreational	1.1	2.3	3.4	4.6	5.7
5.4	ping pong	1.9	3.7	5.6	7.4	9.3
14.3	martial arts	0.7	1.4	2.1	2.8	3.5
10.6	swimming laps	0.9	1.9	2.8	3.8	4.7
7	golf (pull, carry clubs)	1.4	2.9	4.3	5.7	7.1
5	pilates	2.0	4.0	6.0	8.0	10.0
3.6	yoga	2.8	5.6	8.3	11.1	13.9
1.75	driving car	5.7	11.4	17.1	22.9	28.6
1.8	lying or sitting quietly	5.6	11.1	16.7	22.2	27.8
2.2	standing quietly	4.5	9.1	13.6	18.2	22.7
2.2	typing on cumputer	4.5	9.1	13.6	18.2	22.7

AT180(cont)

180 pound person
*Number of minutes needed to burn off calories
given in 10 calorie intervals*

60	70	80	90	100	200	300	400
min	min	min	min	min	min	min	min
10.5	12.3	14.0	15.8	17.5	35.1	52.6	70.2
7.3	8.5	9.8	11.0	12.2	24.4	36.6	48.8
8.6	10.0	11.4	12.9	14.3	28.6	42.9	57.1
4.2	4.9	5.6	6.3	7.0	14.0	21.0	28.0
3.0	3.5	4.0	4.5	5.0	9.9	14.9	19.8
11.3	13.2	15.1	17.0	18.9	37.7	56.6	75.5
5.5	6.4	7.3	8.3	9.2	18.3	27.5	36.7
4.9	5.7	6.6	7.4	8.2	16.4	24.6	32.8
6.9	8.0	9.2	10.3	11.5	23.0	34.5	46.0
11.1	13.0	14.8	16.7	18.5	37.0	55.6	74.1
4.2	4.9	5.6	6.3	7.0	14.0	21.0	28.0
5.7	6.6	7.5	8.5	9.4	18.9	28.3	37.7
8.6	10.0	11.4	12.9	14.3	28.6	42.9	57.1
12.0	14.0	16.0	18.0	20.0	40.0	60.0	80.0
16.7	19.4	22.2	25.0	27.8	55.6	83.3	111.1
34.3	40.0	45.7	51.4	57.1	114.3	171.4	228.6
33.3	38.9	44.4	50.0	55.6	111.1	166.7	222.2
27.3	31.8	36.4	40.9	45.5	90.9	136.4	181.8
27.3	31.8	36.4	40.9	45.5	90.9	136.4	181.8

AT200

200 pound person
Number of minutes needed to burn off calories given in 10 calorie intervals

	calorie intervals	10	20	30	40	50
		min	min	min	min	min
cal/min	activities					
6.3	aquaerobics	1.6	3.2	4.8	6.3	7.9
8.9	aerobics, medium	1.1	2.2	3.4	4.5	5.6
7.8	walking 3.5 mph	1.3	2.6	3.8	5.1	6.4
15.6	jogging (6.5 mph)	0.6	1.3	1.9	2.6	3.2
20.8	running (10 mph)	0.5	1.0	1.4	1.9	2.4
5.5	cycling (5.5 mph)	1.8	3.6	5.5	7.3	9.1
11.8	soccer	0.8	1.7	2.5	3.4	4.2
13.5	raquetball	0.7	1.5	2.2	3.0	3.7
9.4	tennis- recreational	1.1	2.1	3.2	4.3	5.3
5.8	ping pong	1.7	3.4	5.2	6.9	8.6
15.6	martial arts	0.6	1.3	1.9	2.6	3.2
11.9	swimming laps	0.8	1.7	2.5	3.4	4.2
7.6	golf (pull, carry clubs)	1.3	2.6	3.9	5.3	6.6
5.6	pilates	1.8	3.6	5.4	7.1	8.9
4	yoga	2.5	5.0	7.5	10.0	12.5
1.8	driving car	5.6	11.1	16.7	22.2	27.8
1.8	lying or sitting quietly	5.6	11.1	16.7	22.2	27.8
2.3	standing quietly	4.3	8.7	13.0	17.4	21.7
2.3	typing on cumputer	4.3	8.7	13.0	17.4	21.7

AT200(cont)

200 pound person

*Number of minutes needed to burn off calories
given in 10 calorie intervals*

60	70	80	90	100	200	300	400
min	min	min	min	min	min	min	min
9.5	11.1	12.7	14.3	15.9	31.7	47.6	63.5
6.7	7.9	9.0	10.1	11.2	22.5	33.7	44.9
7.7	9.0	10.3	11.5	12.8	25.6	38.5	51.3
3.8	4.5	5.1	5.8	6.4	12.8	19.2	25.6
2.9	3.4	3.8	4.3	4.8	9.6	14.4	19.2
10.9	12.7	14.5	16.4	18.2	36.4	54.5	72.7
5.1	5.9	6.8	7.6	8.5	16.9	25.4	33.9
4.4	5.2	5.9	6.7	7.4	14.8	22.2	29.6
6.4	7.4	8.5	9.6	10.6	21.3	31.9	42.6
10.3	12.1	13.8	15.5	17.2	34.5	51.7	69.0
3.8	4.5	5.1	5.8	6.4	12.8	19.2	25.6
5.0	5.9	6.7	7.6	8.4	16.8	25.2	33.6
7.9	9.2	10.5	11.8	13.2	26.3	39.5	52.6
10.7	12.5	14.3	16.1	17.9	35.7	53.6	71.4
15.0	17.5	20.0	22.5	25.0	50.0	75.0	100.0
33.3	38.9	44.4	50.0	55.6	111.1	166.7	222.2
33.3	38.9	44.4	50.0	55.6	111.1	166.7	222.2
26.1	30.4	34.8	39.1	43.5	87.0	130.4	173.9
26.1	30.4	34.8	39.1	43.5	87.0	130.4	173.9

AT220

220 pound person
Number of minutes needed to burn off calories
given in 10 calorie intervals

cal/min	calorie intervals	10 min	20 min	30 min	40 min	50 min
	activities					
6.9	aquaerobics	1.4	2.9	4.3	5.8	7.2
11	aerobics, medium	0.9	1.8	2.7	3.6	4.5
8.6	walking 3.5 mph	1.2	2.3	3.5	4.7	5.8
17.2	jogging (6.5 mph)	0.6	1.2	1.7	2.3	2.9
27.6	running (10 mph)	0.4	0.7	1.1	1.4	1.8
6.38	cycling (5.5 mph)	1.6	3.1	4.7	6.3	7.8
	soccer					
15.2	raquetball	0.7	1.3	2.0	2.6	3.3
	tennis- recreational					
6.82	ping pong	1.5	2.9	4.4	5.9	7.3
17.2	martial arts	0.6	1.2	1.7	2.3	2.9
12.8	swimming laps	0.8	1.6	2.3	3.1	3.9
8.36	golf (pull, carry clubs)	1.2	2.4	3.6	4.8	6.0
6.1	pilates	1.6	3.3	4.9	6.6	8.2
4.3	yoga	2.3	4.7	7.0	9.3	11.6
	driving car					
1.98	lying or sitting quietly	5.1	10.1	15.2	20.2	25.3
	standing quietly					
	typing on cumputer					

AT220(cont)

220 pound person
Number of minutes needed to burn off calories
given in 10 calorie intervals

60	70	80	90	100	200	300	400
min	min	min	min	min	min	min	min
8.7	10.1	11.6	13.0	14.5	29.0	43.5	58.0
5.5	6.4	7.3	8.2	9.1	18.2	27.3	36.4
7.0	8.1	9.3	10.5	11.6	23.3	34.9	46.5
3.5	4.1	4.7	5.2	5.8	11.6	17.4	23.3
2.2	2.5	2.9	3.3	3.6	7.2	10.9	14.5
9.4	11.0	12.5	14.1	15.7	31.3	47.0	62.7
3.9	4.6	5.3	5.9	6.6	13.2	19.7	26.3
8.8	10.3	11.7	13.2	14.7	29.3	44.0	58.7
3.5	4.1	4.7	5.2	5.8	11.6	17.4	23.3
4.7	5.5	6.3	7.0	7.8	15.6	23.4	31.3
7.2	8.4	9.6	10.8	12.0	23.9	35.9	47.8
9.8	11.5	13.1	14.8	16.4	32.8	49.2	65.6
14.0	16.3	18.6	20.9	23.3	46.5	69.8	93.0
30.3	35.4	40.4	45.5	50.5	101.0	151.5	202.0

AT240

240 pound person
Number of minutes needed to burn off calories given in 10 calorie intervals

	calorie intervals	10	20	30	40	50
		min	min	min	min	min
cal/min	activities					
7.6	aquaerobics	1.3	2.6	3.9	5.3	6.6
11	aerobics, medium	0.9	1.8	2.7	3.6	4.5
9.4	walking 3.5 mph	1.1	2.1	3.2	4.3	5.3
19.2	jogging (6.5 mph)	0.5	1.0	1.6	2.1	2.6
27.6	running (10 mph)	0.4	0.7	1.1	1.4	1.8
7	cycling (5.5 mph)	1.4	2.9	4.3	5.7	7.1
	soccer					
16.1	raquetball	0.6	1.2	1.9	2.5	3.1
	tennis- recreational					
7.44	ping pong	1.3	2.7	4.0	5.4	6.7
19.2	martial arts	0.5	1.0	1.6	2.1	2.6
14.3	swimming laps	0.7	1.4	2.1	2.8	3.5
9.12	golf (pull, carry clubs)	1.1	2.2	3.3	4.4	5.5
6.7	pilates	1.5	3.0	4.5	6.0	7.5
4.8	yoga	2.1	4.2	6.3	8.3	10.4
	driving car					
2.16	lying or sitting quietly	4.6	9.3	13.9	18.5	23.1
	standing quietly					
	typing on computer					

AT240(cont)

240 pound person
Number of minutes needed to burn off calories given in 10 calorie intervals

60	70	80	90	100	200	300	400
min	min	min	min	min	min	min	min
7.9	9.2	10.5	11.8	13.2	26.3	39.5	52.6
5.5	6.4	7.3	8.2	9.1	18.2	27.3	36.4
6.4	7.4	8.5	9.6	10.6	21.3	31.9	42.6
3.1	3.6	4.2	4.7	5.2	10.4	15.6	20.8
2.2	2.5	2.9	3.3	3.6	7.2	10.9	14.5
8.6	10.0	11.4	12.9	14.3	28.6	42.9	57.1
3.7	4.3	5.0	5.6	6.2	12.4	18.6	24.8
8.1	9.4	10.8	12.1	13.4	26.9	40.3	53.8
3.1	3.6	4.2	4.7	5.2	10.4	15.6	20.8
4.2	4.9	5.6	6.3	7.0	14.0	21.0	28.0
6.6	7.7	8.8	9.9	11.0	21.9	32.9	43.9
9.0	10.4	11.9	13.4	14.9	29.9	44.8	59.7
12.5	14.6	16.7	18.8	20.8	41.7	62.5	83.3
27.8	32.4	37.0	41.7	46.3	92.6	138.9	185.2

I know I said I wanted to lose weight,
but I'm hungry.

I found an appetite depressant that
really works.

It's called food.

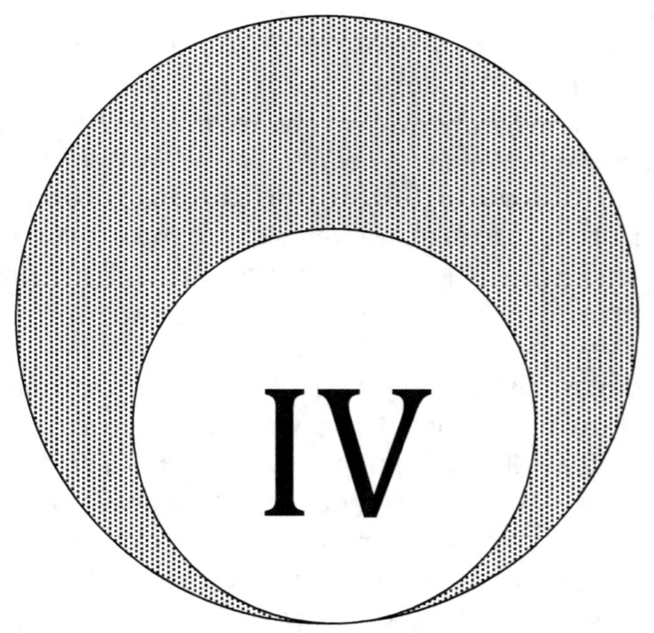

End Notes

Chapter 15

Be Patient and not Paranoid

The trick is to not become paranoid. We should exercise and learn to trust our common sense. We should stop looking out there to science, to doctors, to drugs, to therapies, to our past, our childhood, our environment, for reasons and solutions in weight control. We should admit that no matter how much we know or discover or invent, the one fundamental truth about weight management will remain: eat more calories than you burn and you will gain weight. Unfortunately no one can burn up our calories for us. That is something everyone must do for themselves.

We must also learn to be patient and determined. You didn't gain 10 pounds in a day; you can't lose it in a day. Remember that 3 extra chips over your calorie budget consistently every day will get you 2 pounds in a year. Fortunately all eating waxes and wanes a bit, but if you keep it on the waxing side, you will see the scales go up. (Activity also waxes and wanes. That, however, you do want to keep on the waxing side.)

Eventually we must come to the place where we learn to exercise self discipline in our eating habits as a way of life. Self indulgence has a price tag. Nutrition experts, health centers, athletic clubs, physical fitness experts, food replacements such as nutrasweet, and other gimmicks will not make us thin anywhere except in our pocket books. Let's admit that we like to eat, we like the taste of food. Science came out with sugar substitutes and fat free cookies but did we get thinner? No.

Why not? Because we ate more. Ate more and probably did less. And tormented our bodies along the way.

Eating is our best, most perfect and purest addiction. Because we need to eat and like to eat, we are manipulated and treated like toys. We are jounced like a yo-yo between all those wonderful new foods, gourmet restaurants, tasty snacks that you can take in your car, giant gulp cups on one side, and diet plans, drugs, schemes, and even downright quackery that promise to literally and figuratively balance the scale on the other side.

The fortunate part is that we don't need any of this smorgasbord of pickings to survive. There is no way out except to take charge of our own bodies and mind. We need to find our own way through the maze of temptation and lies, tighten our belts of determination and close the door on the media's larder of manufactured tastes and pleasures and promises.

Make it Way of Life

If you are a little person and would like to eat like a heavy weight boxer, you would soon become a fat person who needs two trips to get all of you to the other side of the room. So exercise discipline every day. It's no different than deciding to read the newspaper before you go to work or say your prayers before you go to bed, or take a walk after supper. It becomes a way of life. It becomes you...and it becomes you. It's way cool. And you will be

WEIGH COOL!

I lost 30 pounds on my reduced joy diet.

A. Watkins

My Final Rant on Calories

Dear Reader,

Calories are not ideas you can spin. You can try to redefine them (soFAS), call them different names (good and empty), even split them up (active and inactive), but that's just a lot of busy work. That's just something for people to do who don't want to face the cold hard truth straight on.

It's not going to help, you know. A calorie is still going to be the amount of energy needed to raise the temperature of one gram of water by one degree Celsius at a pressure of one atmosphere. It's still going to take 3500 of them to burn up 1 pound of fat.

The nicknames for the calories are sometimes misleading. In the English language, empty means containing nothing. Does that mean you can eat lots of empty calories because they don't contain anything? Well actually, no. It means they don't contain much in the way of nutrition or essential vitamins and minerals. They work just the same as nutritional calories. That is, they take just as much energy to burn off. The problem is, they don't contribute to your body's health. For example, alcohol. You can drink martinis all day and only martinis, and the only real food value you will give to your body are the ones found in the olives. Your body needs nutrients, vitamins and minerals to function properly and empty calories give it nothing. You eat 3500 extra empty calories, you gain another pound, but your body didn't get anything out of it. It's like paying your money to see a show, but the screen is black, so you see nothing.

How about the soFAS calories. Again, this is a nickname for the calories that are chocked full of solid fats and added sugars. OK, good idea. Don't eat them. But where are they? They are somewhere in that steak, or that salad dressing, or that peanut butter, etc. Added sugars are in your cereal, in your tomato sauce, in your granola bar. Yikes! They are everywhere! However, unless they are obvious, there is not much you can do about it.

What about active calories and inactive or resting calories? These descriptors come mostly from the sports community. The concept is built into those special watches people buy to keep track of how active they are. Here's how this works. First you get an estimate of how many calories you would burn in a period of time if you did nothing but sit on a couch. They call these "resting calories". So it's not like the calories are resting and as long as you don't wake them up, you can ignore them. Then when you are exercising or even just moving around, the watch's computer converts your movements into the total calories burned. Then the number of "resting calories" is subtracted from the total and this difference refers to the number of "active calories". These are the ones that wouldn't have been burned off if you sat on the couch. Cool.

I say so what? Why should you worry about how they get burned off? It's enough to know that you need to burn off — in some way- all the calories you take in or you will be going into caloric debt. We already talked about how you burn off more calories when you are moving. We also talked about getting the most out our your calories by eating good foods. We talked about how your body needs more than just calories. It needs calories with a balanced set of nutrients to maintain itself properly.

So again, if you want to dicker around with sophisticated definitions, and let them confuse you and make you think weight loss is just too complicated, maybe even make you throw in the towel, I think you should ask yourself if you really want to lose weight anyway. Because burning off more calories than you take in - no matter what you call them, or what kind you think they are, or where you got them - will result in weight loss. Unfortunately the only way you will know if you burned off more than you took in is by being aware of how many you took in and how many you burned off.

I encourage you to be brave, to be patient, and to stay focused on following the rules. God bless you,

Arleen

PS: A little reminder. All those fancy diet plans you buy and follow? They work because they are counting calories for you. And all those tasty foods you buy from them? Those are made with special recipes. And when you make and use your own recipes to make your own pizza and chocolate cake? There's a good chance your recipes will contain a lot more calories. And if they do, guess what will happen then? Bummer.

A. Watkins

What is a Healthy Weight Loss Diet?

A healthy weight loss diet will not only yield results, but will keep your body in great shape physically and nutritionally as well.

A healthy weight loss diet will help you control your calorie intake. The average healthy man or woman needs between 1800 and 2200 calories to survive. A weight loss diet should reduce your calorie intake by no more than 300 to 500 calories a day. Otherwise you'll be getting into starvation or crash diet territory!

A good diet promotes eating fruits, vegetables, nuts, seeds, whole grains, lean proteins, and healthy fats. Any diet that tells you to cut out entire food groups is NOT a healthy diet. On the other hand, a healthy diet will discourage use of sugar, trans fats, processed foods, artificial ingredients, and poor quality foods. It will also discourage eating salty foods and the use of extra salt.

The best and most effective diets are the ones that you can keep for a long time. If your diet relies on foods that are very expensive, hard to find, only available online (supplements, for example), or require a lot of time and effort to prepare, it won't be practical and easy to keep.

Along with your healthy diet, please exercise. If nothing else, at least take regular walks.

What is a Yo-Yo Diet?

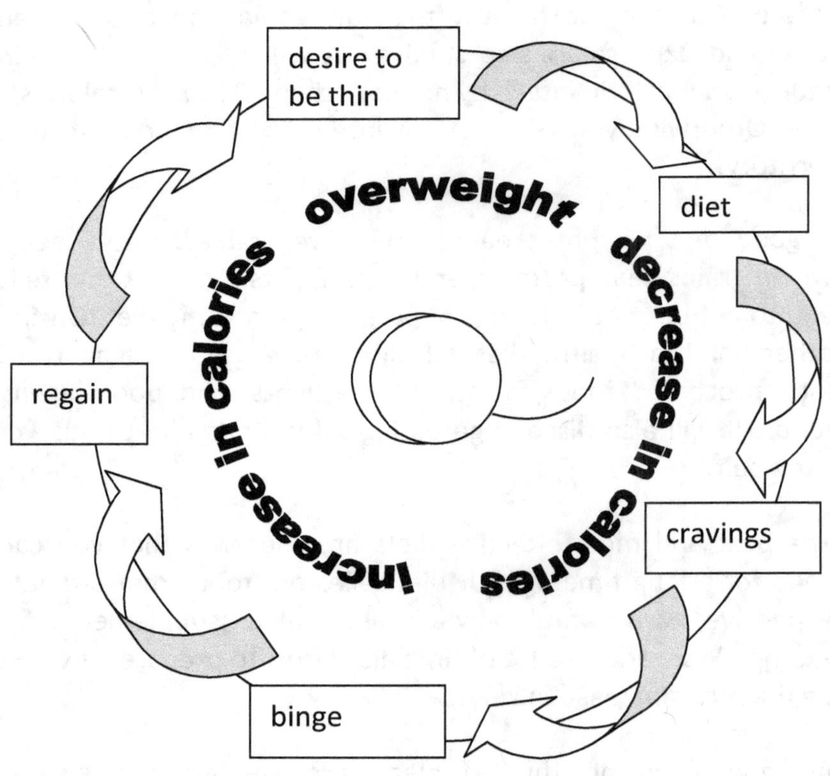

References

About The Author

Dr. Arleen J. Watkins is currently retired. She had been the Director of Curriculum for Family and Community Medicine at the University of Arizona College of Medicine. She was also research associate for AGE WELL, a health promotion program for the elderly, for four years during which she wrote or assisted with several technical papers and authored "Late Bloomers" for <u>American Fitness.</u>

Prior to her position in research with both elderly and medical students, she taught statistics and advanced mathematics at the University of Arizona, University of the Virgin Islands, Pennsylvania State University, University of North Florida and Flagler College. While there, she presented seminars and participated in the writing of many technical papers in the health and science fields.

Her doctorate in measurements and research (applied statistics) and her experiential background in medicine has provided her with knowledge to understand, analyze, and criticize claims of the various diet programs. It has also given her the expertise to create the tables exhibiting the energy relationships between foods and activities used in this book. Her background in research enabled her to investigate and provide the foundation for the claims and ideas put forth in this book.

Calorie Burn Charts

The author looked at hundreds of charts on the internet. While many provided some information, for the most part they did not add new information from the two referenced mostly.

A. Watkins

Direct quotes from these two were not used because neither of them responded to requests for permission. Therefore it is suggested you go to their web sites to get information that may be important or confusing to you. One is a chart copyrighted 2004 by Linda Stradly. Her website is called "What's Cooking America." You can also search on "number of calories burned per minute by exercise and weight." Another chart referenced is by Susan Bowerman. However, her chart did not give enough information about walking speed and terrain and only referred to a 150 pound person. As a result Dr. Watkins used her math and creative skills to combine and convert information from a variety of charts on the internet to construct the tables presented here.